T0269284

Clinicians' Guides to Radionuclide Hybrid Imaging

PET/CT

Series editors
Jamshed B. Bomanji
London, UK

Gopinath Gnanasegaran
London, UK

Stefano Fanti
Bologna, Italy

Homer A.Macapinlac
Houston, Texas, USA

More information about this series at http://www.springer.com/series/13803

Valentina Ambrosini • Stefano Fanti
Editors

PET/CT in Neuroendocrine Tumors

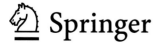

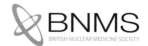

Editors
Valentina Ambrosini
Nuclear Medicine
DIMES University of Bologna,
S.Orsola-Malpighi Hospital
Bologna, Bologna
Italy

Stefano Fanti
Nuclear Medicine
DIMES University of Bologna,
S.Orsola-Malpighi Hospital
Bologna, Bologna
Italy

ISSN 2367-2439   ISSN 2367-2447 (electronic)
Clinicians' Guides to Radionuclide Hybrid Imaging - PET/CT
ISBN 978-3-319-29202-1   ISBN 978-3-319-29203-8 (eBook)
DOI 10.1007/978-3-319-29203-8

Library of Congress Control Number: 2016938547

Printed on acid-free paper

This Springer imprint is published by Springer Nature
The registered company is Springer International Publishing AG Switzerland

Foreword

Clear and concise clinical indications for PET/CT in the management of the oncology patient are presented in this series of 15 separate Booklets.

The impact on better staging, tailored management and specific treatment of the patient with cancer has been achieved with the advent of this multimodality imaging technology. Early and accurate diagnosis will always pay, and clear information can be gathered with PET/CT on treatment responses. Prognostic information is gathered and can forward guide additional therapeutic options.

It is a fortunate coincidence that PET/CT was able to derive great benefit from radionuclide-labelled probes, which deliver good and often excellent target to nontarget signals. Whilst labelled glucose remains the cornerstone for the clinical benefit achieved, a number of recent probes are definitely adding benefit. PET/CT is hence an evolving technology, extending its applications and indications. Significant advances in the instrumentation and data processing available have also contributed to this technology, which delivers high throughput and a wealth of data, with good patient tolerance and indeed patient and public acceptance. As an example, the role of PET/CT in the evaluation of cardiac disease is also covered, with emphasis on labelled rubidium and labelled glucose studies.

The novel probes of labelled choline, labelled peptides, such as DOTATATE, and, most recently, labelled PSMA (prostate-specific membrane antigen) have gained rapid clinical utility and acceptance, as significant PET/CT tools for the management of neuroendocrine disease and prostate cancer patients, notwithstanding all the advances achieved with other imaging modalities, such as MRI. Hence, a chapter reviewing novel PET tracers forms part of this series.

The oncological community has recognised the value of PET/CT and has delivered advanced diagnostic criteria for some of the most important indications for PET/CT. This includes the recent Deauville criteria for the classification of PET/CT patients with lymphoma – similar criteria are expected to develop for other malignancies, such as head and neck cancer, melanoma and pelvic malignancies. For completion, a separate section covers the role of PET/CT in radiotherapy planning, discussing the indications for planning biological tumour volumes in relevant cancers.

These Booklets offer simple, rapid and concise guidelines on the utility of PET/CT in a range of oncological indications. They also deliver a rapid aide memoire on the merits and appropriate indications for PET/CT in oncology.

London, UK   Peter J. Ell, FMedSci, DR HC, AΩA

Preface

Hybrid Imaging with PET/CT and SPECT/CT combines the best of function and structure to provide accurate localisation, characterisation and diagnosis. There is extensive literature and evidence to support PET/CT, which has made significant impact in oncological imaging and management of patients with cancer. The evidence in favour of SPECT/CT especially in orthopaedic indications is evolving and increasing.

The Clinicians' Guides to Radionuclide Hybrid Imaging pocketbook series is specifically aimed at our referring clinicians, nuclear medicine/radiology doctors, radiographers/technologists and nurses who are routinely working in nuclear medicine and participate in multidisciplinary meetings. This series is the joint work of many friends and professionals from different nations who share a common dream and vision towards promoting and supporting nuclear medicine as a useful and important imaging speciality.

We want to thank all those people who have contributed to this work as advisors, authors and reviewers, without whom the book would not have been possible. We want to thank our members from the BNMS (British Nuclear Medicine Society, UK) for their encouragement and support, and we are extremely grateful to Dr Brian Nielly, Charlotte Weston, the BNMS Education Committee and the BNMS council members for their enthusiasm and trust.

Finally, we wish to extend particular gratitude to the industry for their continuous supports towards education and training.

London, UK   Gopinath Gnanasegaran
                                                                   Jamshed Bomanji

Acknowledgements

The series co-ordinators and editors would like to express sincere gratitude to the members of British Nuclear Medicine Society, patients, teachers, colleagues, students and industry and the BNMS Education Committee Members for their continued support and inspiration:

Andy Bradley
Brent Drake
Francis Sundram
James Ballinger
Parthiban Arumugam
Rizwan Syed
Sai Han
Vineet Prakash

Contents

Contributors

Valentina Ambrosini Nuclear Medicine, University of Bologna, S.Orsola-Malpighi Hospital, Bologna, Italy

Andrea Andreone Radiology, University of Bologna, U.O. Radiologia III, S.Orsola-Malpighi Hospital, Bologna, Italy

Andy Bradley Manchester Royal Infirmary, Manchester, UK

Davide Campana Department of Medical and Surgical Sciences, S.Orsola-Malpighi University Hospital, Bologna, Italy

John Dickson University College London Hospitals NHS Foundation Trust, London, UK

Stefano Fanti Nuclear Medicine, University of Bologna, S.Orsola-Malpighi Hospital, Bologna, Italy

Nicola Fazio Unit of Gastrointestinal Medical Oncology and Neuroendocrine Tumours, European Institute of Oncology, Milan, Italy

Margarita Kirienko Nuclear Medicine, Niguarda – Cà Granda Hospital, University Milano Bicocca, Milan, Italy

Mauro Papotti University of Turin at San Luigi Hospital, Orbassano, Italy

Giovanna Pepe Nuclear Medicine, Humanitas Research Hospital, Milan, Italy

Carla Serra Interventional and Diagnostic Ultrasound, S.Orsola-Malpighi Hospital, Bologna, Italy

Francesca Spada Unit of Gastrointestinal Medical Oncology and Neuroendocrine Tumours, European Institute of Oncology, Milan, Italy

Paola Tomassetti Department of Medical and Surgical Sciences, S.Orsola-Malpighi University Hospital, Bologna, Italy

Deborah Tout Gold Coast University Hospital, Southport, QLD, Australia

Marco Volante University of Turin at San Luigi Hospital, Orbassano, Italy

Incidence, Epidemiology, Aetiology and Staging, Classification, Clinical Presentation/Signs and Symptoms, Diagnosis, Staging Procedures/ Investigation

1

Davide Campana and Paola Tomassetti

Contents

1.1   Incidence, Epidemiology

Neuroendocrine tumours (NET) comprise a large variety of rare and heterogeneous tumours with an estimated incidence of 3–5/100,000/year. They can arise in virtually every internal organ, but mainly occur in the gastroenteropancreatic and bronchopulmonary systems. Gastrointestinal and pancreatic neuroendocrine tumours (GEP-NET) include various types of solid tumours arising from the secretory cells of the neuroendocrine cell system; they can occur anywhere along the gastrointestinal tract.

In the past, these tumours have been considered rare diseases, although the most recent data from the US Surveillance Epidemiology and End Results (SEER) program show an impressive increase in the incidence of this disease (520 %) over the past 32 years (1973–2005), with an annual percentage increase of 5.8 % [1–9]. The incidence, from 1.1 per 100,000 people in 1973, reached 6.2 per 100,000 people in 2005. Much of this increase probably reflects the introduction of more sensitive diagnostic tools as well as an increased awareness among physicians.

D. Campana (✉) • P. Tomassetti
Department of Medical and Surgical Sciences, S.Orsola-Malpighi University Hospital, Bologna, Italy
e-mail: davide.campana@unibo.it

© Springer International Publishing Switzerland 2016   1
V. Ambrosini, S. Fanti (eds.), *PET/CT in Neuroendocrine Tumors*,
Clinicians' Guides to Radionuclide Hybrid Imaging: PET/CT,
DOI 10.1007/978-3-319-29203-8_1

According to the SEER program, the incidence of these tumours was estimated to be approximately 35/100,000 in 2004. Given the overall slow growth of these tumours, the prevalence renders GEP-NET the second most common gastrointestinal cancer after colon cancer.

Gastrointestinal and pancreatic neuroendocrine tumours are most common in the small intestine (30.8 %), followed by the rectum (26.3 %), colon (17.6 %), pancreas (12.1 %), stomach (8.9 %) and appendix (5.7 %). Around 25 % of the NET are localised in the bronchopulmonary system.

The prognosis of GEP-NET patients is good when compared to adenocarcinomas in the same location. The 5-year survival rates are highest in rectal and appendiceal NET, but lower in small intestinal and pancreatic NET, with notable variability in survival between countries in Europe and the USA.

The survival of patients with GEP-NET depends on stage and histology. Data from the SEER database show an important improvement in survival in recent years (1998–2004).

1.2   Aetiology and Staging, Classification

Gastrointestinal and pancreatic neuroendocrine tumours usually arise sporadically; however, they can be the result of hereditary predisposition syndromes, such as multiple endocrine neoplasia type 1, Von Hippel-Lindau's disease or neurofibromatosis type 1.

These tumours have traditionally been divided into foregut (oesophagus, stomach, proximal duodenum, liver and pancreas), midgut (distal duodenum ileum, jejunum, ascending colon and the proximal two-thirds of the transverse colon) and hindgut (distal third of the transverse colon, descending colon, sigmoid colon and rectum) tumours.

The WHO 2010 classification adopts the definition NET (neuroendocrine tumour) for low-to-intermediate-grade tumours (G1, G2) and NEC (neuroendocrine carcinoma) for high-grade tumours (G3) referring to Ki-67 or MIB-1 (Table 1.1). Staging is adopted as an important instrument for patient stratification and is carried out according to site-specific tumour-node-metastasis (TNM) classification (ENET [European Neuroendocrine Tumour Society] or AJCC [American Joint Committee

Table 1.1 The 2010 WHO classification for NET

Classification	Grading		
	Grade	MIB-1 – mitotic count (per 10 HPF)[a]	Ki-67 index (%)[b]
NET	G1	<2	≤2
NET	G2	2–20	3–20
NEC	G3	>20	>20

Abbreviations: *NET* neuroendocrine tumour, *NEC* neuroendocrine carcinoma
[a]10 HPF: high-power field = 2 mm², counted in at least 40 fields (at 40× magnification) evaluated in areas of highest mitotic density
[b]Ki-67 index: % of 2000 tumour cells in areas of highest nuclear labelling

on Cancer]). According to the WHO classification of lung tumours, bronchopulmonary NET are subdivided into typical carcinoids (TCs), atypical carcinoids (ACs), large-cell poorly differentiated (LCNEC) and small-cell poorly differentiated (SCLC) neuroendocrine carcinomas.

1.3   Clinical Presentation/Signs and Symptoms

Gastrointestinal and pancreatic neuroendocrine tumours are characterised by their ability to produce, store and secrete a large number of peptide hormones and biogenic amines, which can lead to the development of distinct clinical syndromes. Based on this, GEP-NET can be subdivided into "functioning" or "non-functioning". Functioning tumours are associated with hormonal hypersecretion and determine a clinical syndrome (including carcinoid, Zollinger-Ellison syndrome (ZES), insulinoma, Verner-Morrison and glucagonoma) (Table 1.2). Non-functioning NETs are not associated with a distinct hormonal syndrome; however, non-functioning GEP-NET may also secrete bioactive amines at subclinical levels or secrete compounds which lead to other, still under-recognised hormonal syndromes.

Non-functioning tumours are more difficult to detect than functioning ones. The patients generally present late with large primary tumours and advanced disease, with symptoms of mass effects or distant (usually hepatic) metastasis.

A delayed diagnosis is typical (5–7 years on average), increasing the probability of metastatic disease.

Gastric carcinoids are typically multiple, small, localised tumours associated with hypergastrinaemia, either secondary to chronic atrophic gastritis (type 1) or as part of Zollinger-Ellison syndrome (type 2). These tumours are rarely malignant and have a less than 2–5 % rate of metastasis. On the contrary, large solitary gastric carcinoids (type 3) are not associated with hypergastrinaemia and commonly metastasise. The majority of duodenal NETs are gastrin secreting, causing Zollinger-Ellison syndrome and occurring in patients with MEN1.

Table 1.2   Gastroenteropancreatic neuroendocrine tumours and clinical features

Tumour	Hormone produced	Signs or symptoms
Insulinoma	Insulin, proinsulin	Hypoglycaemic symptoms
Gastrinoma	Gastrin	Abdominal pain, peptic ulcers, oesophageal symptoms, diarrhoea
Glucagonoma	Glucagon	Diabetes/glucose intolerance, necrolytic migratory erythema, weight loss
VIPoma	Vasointestinal polypeptide	Severe watery diarrhoea, hypokalaemia
Intestinal carcinoids	Serotonin	Flushing, diarrhoea, abdominal pain, cardiac fibrosis
Non-functioning tumours	–	Abdominal pain, mass effect, aspecific symptoms

Small intestinal NET are mostly non-functioning. They originate in the distal jejunum and ileum and commonly metastasise to the liver. A typical carcinoid syndrome occurs in approximately 18% of cases. This syndrome is related to the presence of liver metastases; in these patients, serotonin, tachykinins and other bioactive substances can reach the systemic circulation and cause carcinoid syndrome, characterised by cutaneous flushing, diarrhoea and abdominal pain. Moreover, liver involvement from metastatic disease might cause symptoms related to tumour bulk and capsular invasion. A distinct feature of NET is their propensity to cause extensive mesenteric fibrosis and, occasionally, mesenteric ischaemia. Fibrosis might involve the endocardium of the right side of the heart, and the tricuspid and pulmonary valves, with impairment of cardiac function. Ten to 20% of patients with carcinoid syndrome have heart disease at presentation.

Appendiceal carcinoids are usually confined to the appendix and are identified incidentally during unrelated surgery or during acute appendicitis.

Neuroendocrine tumours of the colon are large tumours and have the poorest prognosis of all GEP-NET; patients commonly present with liver metastases.

Rectal carcinoids are usually diagnosed incidentally during colonoscopy and are typically small, localised, non-functioning tumours which rarely metastasise (perhaps owing to early detection).

A huge proportion of the bronchopulmonary NET are asymptomatic at initial diagnosis. In other cases, they appear with cough, hemoptysis and bronchopulmonary infections. They also can occur with carcinoid syndrome.

The majority of pancreatic NET are large, up to 40% are non-functioning and approximately 50% have hepatic metastasis at diagnosis. Functioning pancreatic NET may secrete several peptide hormones and lead to diverse symptomatologies. Insulinomas are typically small, benign, functioning tumours which present with hypoglycaemia. Pancreatic gastrinomas are less common than duodenal gastrinomas, but are usually malignant; approximately 25% are associated with MEN1. Glucagonomas, which cause diabetes and a characteristic rash (necrolytic migratory erythema), and VIPomas, which are associated with severe diarrhoea, are large tumours which have already metastasised when diagnosed. Other rare functioning tumours which secrete adrenocorticotropic hormone, growth hormone-releasing hormone, parathyroid hormone-related protein and somatostatin have been reported. They may be difficult to diagnose because of intermittent peptide release, unusual symptoms and fluctuating plasma hormone levels.

1.4   Diagnosis, Staging Procedures/Investigation

The diagnosis of NET is multimodal, based on clinical symptoms, hormone levels, radiological and nuclear imaging and histological confirmation. An early accurate diagnosis is often delayed as most NET are small, initially asymptomatic and non-functioning.

The most important general tumour marker is chromogranin A (CgA), expressed in 80–90% of all patients with NET, and is correlated with tumour mass. Another general marker is neuron-specific enolase (NSE), especially expressed in NECs of the lung. Among functioning tumours, specific markers are 5-hydroxindoleacetic acid (5-HIAA), insulin, gastrin, glucagon and vasoactive intestinal polypeptide (VIP).

Imaging modalities for diagnosis and staging include conventional radiology, such as transabdominal ultrasonography, endoscopic ultrasonography, computed tomography (CT), magnetic resonance imaging (MRI) and nuclear imaging, including somatostatin receptor scintigraphy (octreoscan) or positron emission tomography (PET) with (68)Ga-DOTA-peptides, the latter having a very elevated sensitivity.

Key Points
- Neuroendocrine tumours (NET) comprise a large variety of rare and heterogeneous tumours with an estimated incidence of 3–5/100,000/year.
- The diagnosis of NET is multimodal, based on clinical symptoms, hormone levels, radiological and nuclear imaging and histological confirmation.
- The survival of patients with GEP-NET depends on stage and histology.
- The 5-year survival rates are highest in rectal and appendiceal NET.
- Neuroendocrine tumours of the colon are large tumours and have the poorest prognosis of all GEP-NET.

References

1. Yao JC, Hassan M, Phan A, Dagohoy C, Leary C, Mares JE, Abdalla EK, Fleming JB, Vauthey JN, Rashid A, et al. One hundred years after "carcinoid": epidemiology of and prognostic factors for neuroendocrine tumors in 35,825 cases in the United States. J Clin Oncol. 2008;26:3063–72.
2. Bosman FT, Carneiro F, Hruban RH, Theise ND, editors. WHO classification of tumours of the digestive system, vol. 3. 4th ed. Lyon: IARC Press; 2010.
3. Sobin LH, Gospodarowicz MK, Wittekind C, editors. TNM classification of malignant tumours. 7th ed. Chichester: Wiley-Blackwell; 2009.
4. Edge SB, et al., editors. AJCC cancer staging manual. 7th ed. New York: Springer; 2010.
5. Hörsch D, Schmid KW, Anlauf M, Darwiche K, Denecke T, Baum RP, Spitzweg C, Grohé C, Presselt N, Stremmel C, Heigener DF, Serke M, Kegel T, Pavel M, Waller CF, Deppermann KM, Arnold R, Huber RM, Weber MM, Hoffmann H. Neuroendocrine tumors of the bronchopulmonary system (typical and atypical carcinoid tumors): current strategies in diagnosis and treatment. Oncol Res Treat. 2014;37(5):266–76.
6. Modlin IM, Kidd M, Latich I, et al. Current status of gastrointestinal carcinoids. Gastroenterology. 2005;128:1717–51.
7. Kaltsas GA, Besser GM, Grossman AB. The diagnosis and medical management of advanced neuroendocrine tumors. Endocr Rev. 2004;25:458–511.
8. Modlin IM, et al. Gastrointestinal neuroendocrine (carcinoid) tumours: current diagnosis and management. Med J Aust. 2010;193:46–52.
9. Ambrosini V, Tomassetti P, Franchi R, Fanti S. Imaging of NET with PET radiopharmaceuticals. Q J Nucl Med Mol Imaging. 2010;54:16–23.

Pathology of Neuroendocrine Tumors

2

Marco Volante and Mauro Papotti

Contents

2.1 Histological Classification and Features

A spectrum of neuroendocrine (NE) neoplasms (NENs) exists, including well differentiated (generally low grade) tumors and the highly aggressive poorly differentiated small and large cell carcinomas. The latter are relatively homogeneous tumors in different organs and recapitulate the more common pulmonary counterparts. Well differentiated neoplasms occur more commonly in the gastroenteropancreatic (GEP) area, lung, and thymus, either as sporadic forms or in the setting of inherited tumor syndromes. These tumors are however differently classified and labeled. Precursor lesions have been identified (as microscopic findings only), including NE cell hyperplasia and "microcarcinoids" in the stomach and lung (in the latter termed tumorlets, defined as peribronchial NETs having a size not exceeding 5 mm).

The classification of gastroenteropancreatic NENs has undergone major changes in the last edition of the WHO classification of digestive tract tumors [1] (Table 2.1). Although all NETs were considered potentially malignant, the proposal was made to restrict the term "NE carcinoma" to high-grade tumors, only: these were formerly

M. Volante (✉)
Department of Pathology, University of Turin at San Luigi Hospital, Orbassano, Italy
e-mail: marco.volante@unito.it

M. Papotti
Department of Pathology, University of Turin at Città Della Salute Hospital, Turin, Italy

© Springer International Publishing Switzerland 2016
V. Ambrosini, S. Fanti (eds.), *PET/CT in Neuroendocrine Tumors*,
Clinicians' Guides to Radionuclide Hybrid Imaging: PET/CT,
DOI 10.1007/978-3-319-29203-8_2

Table 2.1 Comparative scheme of different WHO classifications of NET

Type of NET	Well diff.	Moderately diff.	Poorly differentiated	Mixed
GEP-NET				
WHO 2000	WD NET	WD NEC	PD NEC (small/large cells)	MEEC
WHO 2010	NET G1	NET G2	NEC (small/large cells) (G3)	MANEC
Lung				
WHO 2004	Typical carcinoid	Atypical carcinoid	Small cell lung carcinoma Large cell NE carcinoma	Combined Carcinoma

Abbreviations: *NET* neuroendocrine tumor, *diff* differentiated, *GEP* gastroenteropancreatic, *NEC* neuroendocrine carcinoma, *MEEC* mixed exocrine-endocrine carcinoma, *MANEC* mixed adeno-neuroendocrine carcinoma, *NE* neuroendocrine, *G* tumor grade [G1, <2 mitoses/10 HPF and/or ≤2 % Ki-67; G2, 2–20 mitoses/10 HPF and/or 3–20 % Ki-67; G3, >20 mitoses/10 HPF and/or >20 % Ki-67]

identified as poorly differentiated NE carcinomas (or PDCA). Currently, these neoplasms are called NE carcinomas, morphologically resemble small or large cell cancers of the lung, and are by default grade 3 tumors (i.e., having >20 mitoses per 10 high-power fields and a Ki-67 index >20 %). They are more commonly encountered in the stomach and colorectum and more rarely in the pancreas. On the other side of the spectrum, well differentiated forms of NE neoplasms (i.e., "carcinoids" of the old terminology) are incorporated under the umbrella term NET, and a grading is necessarily associated, to take low-grade tumors (G1: <2 mitoses per 10 high-power fields and a Ki-67 index ≤2 %) apart from intermediate-grade NETs (G2: 2–20 mitoses per 10 high-power fields and a Ki-67 index in range 3–20 %) (Fig. 2.1). NETs (i.e., well differentiated forms) may rarely be graded as G3 based on their high proliferative activity. Recent data indicate that such tumors have an organoid architecture resembling well differentiated NETs, have a higher proliferative potential, and follow a clinical course intermediate between low-grade NETs and high-grade NE carcinomas [10]. Finally, a staging system was also introduced to identify the extent of invasion, using different criteria in the different locations, including depth of invasion, and the presence of nodal or distant metastases [6].

Conversely, the classification of lung NETs did not change in the last decade and still combines architectural patterns (e.g., organoid growth versus small cell diffuse growth) with the mitotic index and the presence of necrosis, for the purpose of recognizing the four different categories proposed in the spectrum of pure lung NETs [8] (Fig. 2.2). These include typical carcinoid (TC) [organoid, trabecular, acinar growth, no necrosis, and mitotic count <2×10 high-power fields], atypical carcinoid (AC) [organoid, trabecular, acinar growth, presence of necrosis, and/or mitotic count 2–10×10 high-power fields], and large cell NE carcinomas (LCNEC) [organoid or diffuse growth, extensive necrosis, and mitotic index >10 per 10 high-power fields]. In the 2004 WHO classification of lung tumors, LCNEC was included in the large cell carcinoma category, generally encompassing non-endocrine carcinoma subtypes and having nothing in common with LCNEC, with the possible exception of cell size. NE marker expression (chromogranin and synaptophysin among others) may assist in the differential diagnosis. Finally, small cell lung carcinoma (SCLC)

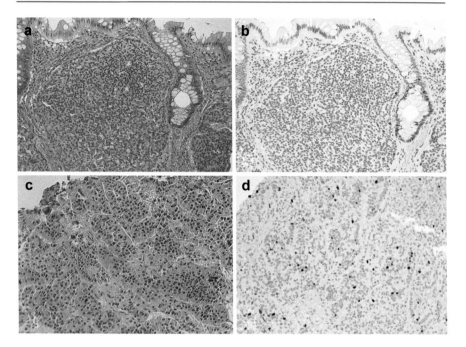

Fig. 2.1 A case of rectal neuroendocrine tumor (**a**), G1 (Ki-67 index <1 %, **b**), which progressed to the liver 2 years later showing a preserved organoid structure (**c**) but increased proliferation (Ki-67 index up to 15 %, **d**)

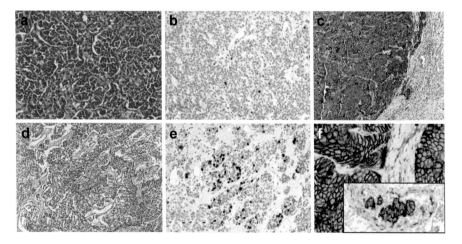

Fig. 2.2 Lung carcinoid tumors. Typical carcinoid is characterized by small cells arranged in nests or trabeculae (**a**) with low Ki-67 index (**b**) and neuroendocrine marker expression, such as chromogranin A (**c**); atypical carcinoid usually grows in a more organoid pattern with focal necrosis (**d**; necrotic areas in the middle of figure), shows an increased Ki-67 index (**e**), and maintains strong expression of SSTR2A (**f**; neoplastic emboli strongly positive for SSTR2A are shown in the *inset*)

is the most common and renowned high-grade pulmonary NE tumor, generally associated to a classical morphology, with few diagnostic problems [3, 8, 9].

In all locations, complex tumors having NE (small and large cell carcinomas) and non-NE (squamous cell or adenocarcinomas) features have been described under the term mixed (for GEP tract) adeno-NE carcinoma (MANEC); they represent a potential diagnostic pitfall in small biopsies and cytology samples. Former mixed appendiceal goblet cell carcinoids are now classified as mucinous adenocarcinomas. In the lung, such tumors are classified as "combined" variants of small and large cell NE carcinoma.

2.1.1 Ki-67 in Lung Neuroendocrine Neoplasms

As outlined above, the Ki-67 proliferative index is necessarily included in the GEP-NET classification, while the histological typing of lung NETs is based on morphology alone. Nevertheless, several data exist in the literature analyzing the prognostic role of Ki-67 in lung NEN definition. It was found that a cutoff of approximately 4% is also a discriminating value for TC versus AC, a figure also accepted for GEP-NET distinction in G1 and G2 tumors (indeed the current WHO classification accepts a 3% cutoff, but recent data indicate that in the pancreatic location, 5% is a more accurate threshold, definitely supporting the notion that well differentiated NENs of different locations are similar tumors with an overlapping proliferative potential). A recent study on lung neuroendocrine tumors suggested to combine morphological parameters (mitoses and necrosis) with Ki-67 index (using specifically settled cutoff values), in order to define a grading system with prognostic validity [2, 7].

2.1.2 Tumor Profiling for Therapeutic Purposes

Novel therapeutic strategies may take advantage from the determination of target molecule expression levels of chemotherapeutic agents (e.g., thymidylate synthase) or oncogenes (e.g., c-Met, EGFR, VEGFR, etc.) which are novel candidate therapeutic targets. Somatostatin receptors (SSTRs) have been identified in NE tumors, including pancreatic and lung NETs. A progressive decrease of SSTR type 2 and 3 reactivity from well (TC, AC) toward poorly differentiated (LCNEC and resected SCLC) forms was observed in lung NE tumors. A correlation with octreotide scintigraphy data was seen in up to 70% of cases [4]. In lung NETs, a lower expression of

Key Points (Table 2.2)
- Neuroendocrine tumor, NET, and carcinoid are synonyms, indicating a well differentiated neoplasm with neuroendocrine differentiation, usually low to intermediate grade.
- Small cell carcinoma, large cell neuroendocrine carcinoma, and neuroendocrine carcinoma are terms indicating a poorly differentiated carcinoma with neuroendocrine features, generally associated to high-grade features and an aggressive behavior.

Table 2.2 Stepwise diagnostic pathology algorithm for neuroendocrine tumors

Define *histological type* based on a 2-tier (gastroenteropancreatic tract) or 4-tier (lung, thymus) system →
Define tumor *grade*, including Ki-67 index (in the gastroenteropancreatic tract) →
Assess tumor *stage* (ENETS and/or AJCC or IASLC) →
Define the *hormonal* production, if any →
Identify pathological parameters of aggressiveness or *prognostic factors, if relevant* →
Screen for *hereditary diseases* (MEN1, VHL, NF1, etc.) *if appropriate* →
Upon request, assess *predictive factors* useful for targeted therapies (e.g. somatostatin receptors, mTOR pathway molecules, thymidylate synthase, other target enzymes, oncoproteins, others)

- Tumor grading and staging are crucial to better characterize a neuroendocrine neoplasm irrespective of its location.
- Immunophenotypic profiling includes diagnostic markers (chromogranin A, synaptophysin, CD56, neurofilaments, and individual hormones according to the site), prognostic markers (namely, Ki-67 proliferation index), and predictive markers of response to therapy (e.g., somatostatin receptors, mTOR pathway molecules, vascular targets of antiangiogenic drugs, etc).
- Genetic tests may be recommended in specific contexts, to define the presence of mutations associated to hereditary diseases (e.g., MEN1, VHL, NF2, etc.).

mTOR was seen in high-grade carcinomas compared to carcinoid tumors, and activated mTOR pathway was correlated with response to mTOR inhibitors in vitro [5].

References

1. Bosman F, Carneiro F, Hruban R, Theise ND. WHO classification of tumours of the digestive system. Lyon: IARC Press; 2010.
2. Pelosi G, Rindi G, Travis WD, Papotti M. Ki-67 antigen in lung neuroendocrine tumors: unraveling a role in clinical practice. J Thorac Oncol. 2014;9(3):273–84.
3. Rekhtman N. Neuroendocrine tumors of the lung: an update. Arch Pathol Lab Med. 2010;134:1628–38.
4. Righi L, Volante M, Tavaglione V, et al. Somatostatin receptor tissue distribution in lung neuroendocrine tumours: a clinicopathologic and immunohistochemical study of 218 'clinically aggressive' cases. Ann Oncol. 2010;21:548–55.
5. Righi L, Volante M, Rapa I, et al. Mammalian target of rapamycin signaling activation patterns in neuroendocrine tumors of the lung. Endocr Relat Cancer. 2010;17:977–87.
6. Rindi G, Falconi M, Klersy C, Albarello L, Boninsegna L, Buchler MW, Capella C, Caplin M, Couvelard A, Doglioni C, Delle Fave G, Fischer L, Fusai G, de Herder WW, Jann H, Komminoth P, de Krijger RR, La Rosa S, Luong TV, Pape U, Perren A, Ruszniewski P, Scarpa

A, Schmitt A, Solcia E, Wiedenmann B. TNM staging of neoplasms of the endocrine pancreas: results from a large international color study. J Natl Cancer Inst. 2012;104(10):764–77.

7. Rindi G, Klersy C, Inzani F, Fellegara G, Ampollini L, Ardizzoni A, Campanini N, Carbognani P, De Pas TM, Galetta D, Granone PL, Righi L, Rusca M, Spaggiari L, Tiseo M, Viale G, Volante M, Papotti M, Pelosi G. Grading the neuroendocrine tumors of the lung: an evidence-based proposal. Endocr Relat Cancer. 2013;21(1):1–16.

8. Travis WD, Brambilla E, Muller-Hermelink HK, Harris CC, World Health Organization Classification of Tumors. Pathology and genetics. Tumours of the lung, pleura, thymus, and heart. Lyon: IARC Press; 2004. p. 31–62.

9. Travis WD, Giroux DJ, Chansky K, et al. The IASLC Lung Cancer Staging Project: proposals for the inclusion of broncho-pulmonary carcinoid tumors in the forthcoming (seventh) edition of the TNM Classification for Lung Cancer. J Thorac Oncol. 2008;3(11):1213–23.

10. Vélayoudom-Céphise FL, Duvillard P, Foucan L, Hadoux J, Chougnet CN, Lebouleux S, Malka D, Guigay J, Goere D, Debaere T, Caramella C, Schlumberger M, Planchard D, Elias D, Ducreux M, Scoazec JY, Baudin E. Are G3 ENETS neuroendocrine neoplasms heterogeneous? Endocr Relat Cancer. 2013;20(5):649–57.

Management of Neuroendocrine Tumors

Nicola Fazio and Francesca Spada

Contents

In neuroendocrine neoplasms (NENs), radical surgical resection represents the only really curative treatment in patients with resectable locally advanced disease.

In the advanced stage, several different therapies can be considered, including medical therapies, peptide radioreceptor therapy (PRRT), and locoregional treatments. Therapeutic approach can change according to the grade of malignancy.

For advanced low-/intermediate-grade NENs, which are the majority of cases, a number of different medical therapies can be considered, including somatostatin analogs (SSAs), interferon (IFN), several chemotherapeutics, and molecular-targeted agents (MTAs) (Fig. 3.1).

Therapeutic options for patients with NENs have been increasing over the years. However, very few therapies were approved for specific settings. Streptozotocin was approved in 1982 by the US Food and Drug Administration (FDA) for patients with advanced pancreatic NENs (PNENs). Octreotide and lanreotide, the two "cold" SSAs commonly used in clinical practice, were approved for treatment of functioning NENs in many countries and are recommended for treatment of progressing nonfunctioning low-grade NENs [1]. In 2011, everolimus, an mTOR inhibitor, and sunitinib, an anti-angiogenic multitargeted inhibitor, were approved by the FDA and then by the European Medicines Agency (EMA) for patients with well/moderately differentiated, progressing,

N. Fazio (✉) • F. Spada
Unit of Gastrointestinal Medical Oncology and Neuroendocrine Tumours,
European Institute of Oncology, Milan, Italy
e-mail: nicola.fazio@ieo.it

© Springer International Publishing Switzerland 2016
V. Ambrosini, S. Fanti (eds.), *PET/CT in Neuroendocrine Tumors*,
Clinicians' Guides to Radionuclide Hybrid Imaging: PET/CT,
DOI 10.1007/978-3-319-29203-8_3

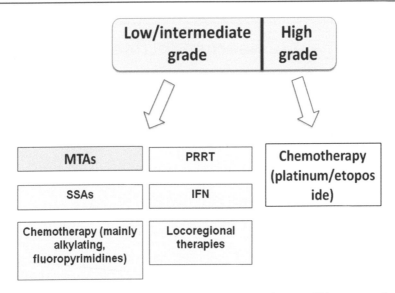

Fig. 3.1 Different treatments in NENs. *MTAs* molecular-targeted agents, *SSAs* somatostatin analogs, *IFN* interferon, *PRRT* peptide radioreceptor therapy

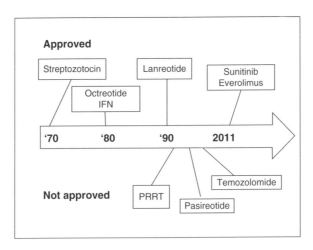

Fig. 3.2 Approved and not approved therapies in NENs. *IFN* interferon, *PRRT* peptide radioreceptor therapy

advanced PNENs. Interferon was approved in some countries for carcinoid syndrome resistant to SSA (Fig. 3.2).

Over the last decade, several prospective randomized large phase III trials were conducted. Two of them included the two SSAs, octreotide long-acting repeatable (LAR) in the PROMID trial [2], and lanreotide autogel in the CLARINET trial [3]. The former, which was published, showed significant progression-free survival (PFS) advantage for octreotide LAR versus placebo in patients with advanced functioning and nonfunctioning midgut NENs with a very low Ki-67 as a first-line treatment. The latter, showed a significant benefit of lanreotide autogel versus placebo in patients with advanced nonfunctioning enteropancreatic NENs, most of them with stable disease at study entry according to RECIST criteria and all with < 10% Ki-67. Based on these two studies, and also on a number of retrospective analyses, octreotide and lanreotide are commonly used in functioning and nonfunctioning, small-bowel and non-small-bowel, progressing and non-progressing NENs and as a first-line and over first-line therapy. However, they should be limited to NENs which are slow growing and with a low proliferation index. Cholelithiasis, diarrhea, bradycardia, hyperglycemia, and hypothyroidism are the most frequent late adverse events.

Everolimus and sunitinib were approved on the basis of results of two placebo-controlled phase III trials in patients with pancreatic well/moderately differentiated, advanced NENs, with a baseline radiological progression. The everolimus trial [4] was completed, with 410 patients, whereas the sunitinib [5] trial was prematurely stopped due to a positive interim analysis. Both trials showed a PFS advantage of around 6 months (5 vs. 11 months in favor of the experimental arm) (Fig. 3.3).

Considering the overall number of patients who received everolimus in the RADIANT-2 [6] and RADIANT-3 [4] trials (419 patients, 215 of them receiving also OCT LAR), the most common all-grade toxicity was aphthous stomatitis (52 %), followed by diarrhea (50 %) and skin rash (47 %). Toxicities more specific

	Experimental arm	Control arm	target	tumors	N° of pts	Author
PROMID	Octreotide LAR	placebo	SSTR-2	Functioning midgut	84	Rinke, JCO 2010
CLARINET	Lanreotide autogel	placebo	SSTR-2	Non-functioning enteropancreatic	204	Caplin, ENETS 2014
RADIANT-3	Everolimus +/- octreotide LAR	Placebo +/- octreotide LAR	mTORC1	PNET	410	Yao, NEJM 2011
A6181111	Sunitinib	placebo	VEGFR, PDGFR, KIT, FLT3, RET	PNET	171	Raymond, NEJM 2011

Fig. 3.3 Randomized phase III trials with SSAs and MTAs in low-/intermediate-grade NENs. *LAR* long-acting repeatable, *SSTR* somatostatin receptor, *mTORC* mammalian target of rapamycin, *PNET* pancreatic neuroendocrine tumor, *VEGFR* vascular endothelial growth factor receptor, *PDGFR* platelet-derived growth factor receptor, *KIT* mast/stem cell growth factor receptor, *FLT* FMS-like tyrosine kinase, *RET* rearranged during transfection gene

for everolimus were hyperglycemia (19 %) and noninfectious pneumonitis (9 %). Grade 3–4 toxicities occurred in less than 5 % of patients, including infections, anemia, hyperglycemia, stomatitis, thrombocytopenia, diarrhea, hypophosphatemia, and neutropenia. Common causes of interruption of everolimus therapy and/or dose reduction were infections, hyperglycemia, noninfectious pneumonitis, and fatigue. Very recently the results of another large phase III trials comparing everolimus with placebo was published. This is the RADIANT-4 trial, which enrolled patients with advanced gastrointestinal, lung and unknown primary well differentiated NENs, all of them with radiological progression at study entry. An around 7 month PFS improvement was obtained in favor of everolimus. Based on that everolimus was approved by FDA for lung and gastrointestinal well differentiated advanced NENs. (Yao et al., Lancet Dec 2015)

The most common adverse events (AEs) associated with sunitinib were diarrhea, nausea, asthenia, vomiting, and fatigue, each occurring in 30 % or more of patients. The most common treatment-related grade 3–4 AEs reported in >10 % of patients were neutropenia (12 %) and hypertension (10 %). All the others were <10 %, including palmar-plantar erythrodysesthesia (6 %), diarrhea (5 %), asthenia (5 %), abdominal pain (5 %), stomatitis (4 %), and thrombocytopenia (4 %).

Regarding chemotherapeutics, temozolomide (TMZ) is an oral alkylating agent that represents the evolution of the parenteral and more toxic streptozotocin. Literature data have been progressively accumulating over the last years, both as single agent and in combination. It has been reported highly active in pancreatic NENs combined with capecitabine [7]. The main toxicities are gastrointestinal (nausea/vomiting, abdominal pain, diarrhea) and hematological (lymphopenia).

For advanced high-grade NENs, platinum/etoposide chemotherapy represents a sort of standard of care, although it is based on old and small-size studies [8].

Peptide radioreceptor therapy is an interesting investigational therapy for NENs. It has been reported to be active and potentially effective in low-/intermediate-grade SSTR-positive NENs. It was not yet approved in any setting, but a regulatory phase III randomized trial the NETTER-1 trial was conducting comparing ^{177}Lu-DOTATATE with octreotide LAR 60 mg/q4w in advanced midgut NENs progressing on octreotide LAR 30 mg/q4w and highly positive at somatostatin receptor scintigraphy. The preliminary results of this trial, which were presented at the 2015 ESMO meeting, showed a clear and significant improvement of PFS in favor of PRRT compared with octreotide LAR 60 mg/4w. In pancreatic NENs, there is retrospective and phase II prospective evidence of activity and potential efficacy of PRRT with ^{177}Lu-DOTATATE. The largest series is 91 patients with advanced pretreated pancreatic NEN included in the retrospective Dutch analysis of 310 gastroenteropancreatic (GEP) NENs published in the JCO in 2008 [9]. Noteworthy are 40 months of time to progression (TTP) (although related to the global population) and more than 40 % of partial response (PR). However, it should be considered that the tumor status at study entry, the proliferation index, and the concomitant use of SSA were unknown for many patients. Therefore, a possible bias related to a spontaneous selection of better prognosis population cannot be excluded. More reliable could be the phase II trial, where 52 patients were prospectively treated with two schedules of ^{177}Lu-DOTATATE, and

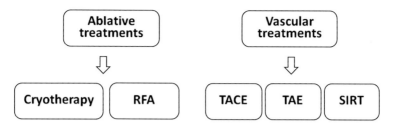

Fig. 3.4 Liver-directed treatments in NENs. *RFA* radiofrequency ablation, *TACE* transarterial chemoembolization, *TAE* transarterial embolization, *SIRT* selective intra-arterial radiotherapy

better results were observed in FDG-PET/CT-negative tumors. A disease control rate (complete response, CR + PR + stable disease, SD) of 80 % with 88 % of tumors progressing at study entry is interesting although also in this case a bias of selection of better prognosis population should be considered [10].

Surgery can have a role also in metastatic NENs, as primary tumor removal and/ or metastasectomy. Even liver orthotopic transplantation can be considered in highly selected patient with very indolent liver-only metastatic NENs. Primary tumor surgical resection is usually considered in small-bowel NENs, with the aim to treat or to prevent an obstructive or bleeding complication. No global agreement exists on the primary tumor removal just to improve prognosis, neither in small-bowel nor in pancreatic NENs. Two recent reviews addressed this point in the two settings leading to no definitive conclusion.

A number of liver-directed treatments have been performed in patients with liver metastases from low-/intermediate-grade NENs. They include ablative treatments such as cryotherapy and radiofrequency ablation and vascular treatments such as transarterial chemoembolization (TACE), embolization (TAE), and selective intra-hepatic radiotherapy (SIRT) (Fig. 3.4).

The former is directed to patients with localized and limited or residual disease (lesions <35 mm in size the latter is performed where a diagnostic superior mesenteric and celiac trunk arteriography is first obtained to evaluate the distribution of hepatic arteries, portal blood flow, and the number and location of hepatic metastases. It causes a vascular occlusion with resulting ischemia to treat hepatic metastases using an emulsion made of cytotoxic drug such as (doxorubicin or STZ).

In patients with diffuse unresectable liver metastases, SIRT could be proposed, and it is performed through the intra-arterial infusion of yttrium-90 (^{90}Y) radiolabeled microsphere.

Conclusion

Over the last years the therapeutic options for NENs have been increased although a standard of therapy or clear criteria of priority for the different medical therapies in the metastatic setting are not established yet.

While the new drugs are currently used in clinical practice, so far we should focus our attention toward a therapeutic strategy based on clinical/biological features of the patient/tumor rather than to a single therapy, and it is possible only within a multidisciplinary team.

Key Points

- In *high-grade advanced* NENs, chemotherapy with platinum and etoposide is the standard first-line therapy, whereas SSAs, MTAs, PRRT, other chemotherapeutics, and locoregional treatments do not have a role. For resistant disease, a second-line chemotherapy, usually camptothecin based, is considered. No particular therapeutic strategy exists.
- In *low/intermediate advanced grade* NENs, different modalities of treatment can have a role and are potentially indicated in the same clinical setting. Due to the poorness of approved standard options, *clinical trials* should be always considered.
- No specific *sequence* of therapies has been validated. *Late toxicity* should be considered when several consecutive systemic therapies are supposed to be used in a patient with a metastatic good-prognosis NEN.
- Presently, no comparative studies have validated a drug or treatment better than any other in the same clinical setting of NENs. Choices should therefore be discussed within a multidisciplinary team based on the patient, tumor, therapy characteristics, evidence, regulatory aspects, and appropriateness.

References

1. Oberg K, Kvols L, Caplin M, et al. Consensus report on the use of somatostatin analogs for the management of neuroendocrine tumors of the gastroenteropancreatic system. Ann Oncol. 2004;15:966–73.
2. Rinke A, Muller HH, Schade-Brittinger C, et al. Placebo-controlled, double-blind, prospective, randomized study on the effect of octreotide LAR in the control of tumor growth in patients with metastatic neuroendocrine midgut tumors: a report from the PROMID study group. J Clin Oncol. 2009;27:4656–63.
3. Caplin M, Phan A, Liyanage N, et al. Lanreotide autogel (depot) significantly improves tumor progression-free survival in patients with non-functioning Gastroenteropancreatic Neuroendocrine Tumors: Results of the CLARINET Study. European Cancer Congress. Abstract 3. Presented 28 Sept 2013; 2013.
4. Yao JC, Shah MH, Ito T, et al. RAD001 in advanced neuroendocrine tumors, third trial (RADIANT-3) study group. Everolimus for advanced pancreatic neuroendocrine tumors. N Engl J Med. 2011;364:514–23.
5. Raymond E, Dahan L, Raoul J-L, et al. Sunitinib malate for the treatment of pancreatic neuroendocrine tumors. N Engl J Med. 2011;364:501–13.
6. Pavel ME, Hainsworth JD, Baudin E. Everolimus plus octreotide long-acting repeatable for the treatment of advanced neuroendocrine tumours associated with carcinoid syndrome (RADIANT-2): a randomised, placebo-controlled, phase 3 study. Lancet. 2011;378(9808):2005–12.
7. Strosberg JR, Fine RL, Choi J, et al. First-line chemotherapy with capecitabine and temozolomide in patients with metastatic pancreatic endocrine carcinomas. Cancer. 2011;117(2):268–75.
8. Moertel CG, Kvols LK, O'Connel MJ. Treatment of neuroendocrine carcinomas with combined etoposide and cisplatin. Cancer. 1991;68:227–32.
9. Kwekkeboom DJ, van de Herder W, Kam BL, et al. Treatment with the radiolabeled somatostatin analog [177Lu-DOTA0, Tyr3] Octreotate: toxicity, efficacy, and survival. J Clin Oncol. 2008;26:2124–30.
10. Sansovini M, Severi S, Ambrosetti A, et al. Treatment with the radiolabelled somatostatin analog Lu-DOTATATE for advanced pancreatic neuroendocrine tumors. Neuroendocrinology. 2013;97(4):347–54.

Imaging of NETs

4

Carla Serra and Andrea Andreone

Contents

4.1 Introduction

Cross-sectional imaging plays an important role for the diagnosis and the staging of neuroendocrine tumors (NETs). Radiological studies are critical to identify the location of the tumor as well as metastases in order to guide appropriate management.

As well as the clinical presentation, imaging findings can be extremely variable [1]. Many neuroendocrine tumors are found through imaging studies performed for other health issues. Diagnosis of functional NETs usually relies upon biochemical and imaging studies, given the smaller size of these tumors, while nonfunctional NETs are more readily detected with radiology.

C. Serra (✉)
Interventional and Diagnostic Ultrasound, S.Orsola-Malpighi Hospital, Bologna, Italy
e-mail: carla.serra@aosp.bo.it

A. Andreone
Radiology, University of Bologna, U.O. Radiologia III, S.Orsola-Malpighi Hospital, Bologna, Italy
e-mail: andrea.andreone1983@gmail.com

© Springer International Publishing Switzerland 2016
V. Ambrosini, S. Fanti (eds.), *PET/CT in Neuroendocrine Tumors*,
Clinicians' Guides to Radionuclide Hybrid Imaging: PET/CT,
DOI 10.1007/978-3-319-29203-8_4

19

4.2   Indications to Radiological Imaging

Imaging studies are performed for three main reasons: to identify the primary lesion, its local extension and relationships with surrounding structures; to assess the TNM staging, therefore to discriminate between surgical and medical therapeutic options; during the follow-up to evaluate radiological response to therapy (restaging) as well as the need for additional treatments [2]. Computed tomography (CT) and magnetic resonance imaging (MRI) are the main imaging modalities employed for detection, staging and treatment response evaluation. Transabdominal ultrasound (US) is usually performed for directing biopsies of the tumoral mass in order to obtain histological diagnosis; on the other hand, contrast-enhanced ultrasound (CEUS) shows high accuracy for the visualization of microvascularization in pancreatic lesions (PNETs) and the detection of liver metastases [3]. Endoscopic ultrasound (EUS) is highly sensitive for the characterization of PNETs and tumors located in the foregut; in addition it allows EUS-guided biopsy of the lesion through fine needle aspiration (EUS-FNA).

4.3   CT

CT is the most used anatomic imaging technique for NET evaluation, due to high spatial resolution, low scan time (especially for what concerns the newest multidetector CT), and an accurate bolus tracking of intravenous (IV) contrast medium.

Patients should be fasted and drink water as an oral contrast agent right before the examination, in order to distend gastric and duodenal walls. An initial precontrast scan is important to detect the primary lesion that can appear as a hypodense area with calcifications (in PNETs and pulmonary NETs). Arterial phase should be started by an accurate bolus tracking of IV contrast or following a delay of 25–30 s after the start of contrast injection. Portal venous phase images should be obtained after a delay of 60–70 s and sometimes can more easily identify the lesion.

NETs are usually hypervascular lesions that enhance during early arterial phase (Fig. 4.1), when the tumor-to-parenchyma contrast is maximized, although the vascular blush is often transient; the delayed portal venous phase usually shows washout of contrast medium.

The detection of small primary tumors of the small bowel is very challenging; therefore the use of a negative oral contrast agent may be helpful. Larger tumors are usually malignant and/or nonfunctioning neoplasms; their typical pattern includes necrosis, calcifications and infiltration of surrounding structures.

CT scan is not recommended in pregnant or lactating women, children, people allergic to iodinated IV contrast media, and nephropathic patients.

Main pitfalls in the use of CT scan are poor ability in the differential diagnosis between small metastatic and reactive lymph nodes and the evidence that Response Evaluation Criteria in Solid Tumors (RECIST) is not sufficient alone to assess response to medical therapy in patients affected by NETs [4].

Detection of the primary tumor depends on size and location: sensitivity range in detecting PNETs is 57–94 %. 85 % of gastrointestinal NETs are visualized through CT enteroclysis, and 44–82 % of liver metastases are detected by CT [5].

Fig. 4.1 CT scan: arterial
phase in coronal view of a
neuroendocrine tumor
located in the head of the
pancreas (*arrows*); it appears
as a hypervascularized lesion
compared to the rest of the
pancreatic gland. * hydropic
gallbladder, # dilated main
bile duct

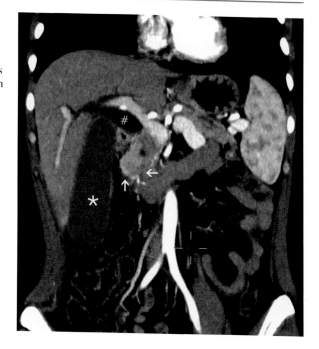

4.4   MRI

MRI study of NETs should be performed on 1.5 or 3 T field strength magnets, including T1-weighted (T1w) and T2-weighted (T2w) sequences with and without fat suppression, diffusion-weighted imaging (DWI), and post-contrast dynamic imaging on arterial, portal venous and delayed phases.

NETs usually appear hypointense on T1w images (Fig. 4.2), while on T2w sequences primary lesions have hyperintense signal; both weighing are more useful when fat suppressed because of the high tumor-to-parenchyma contrast. DWI sequences can be helpful in distinguishing between well- and poorly differentiated NETs, showing the latter lower ADC values probably due to increased tumor cellularity. Post-contrast images show the same features as CT.

MRI has a higher sensitivity than CT in the detection of liver metastases (high signal on T2w sequences, sensitivity 82–95 %) (Fig. 4.3); in particular it has great potential in distinguishing between metastases and benign hepatic lesions especially when performed with hepatocyte- and Kupffer-cell-specific contrast media.

Limitations are those typical of magnetic resonance instrumentation (presence of pacemakers, metallic prosthetic devices, claustrophobia, patient's collaboration, etc).

Main pitfalls are connected to tumor size and to the fact that liver metastases present at diagnosis can be disguised at follow-up examinations, due to fibrotic effects on the liver of medical therapies (chemotherapy, radionuclide therapy, etc.).

Up to 94 % of pancreatic lesions are correctly diagnosed by MRI, while for what concerns primary gastrointestinal NETs, sensitivity of MRI with enteroclysis is 86 % [5].

Fig. 4.2 MRI scan: T1w image showing a hypointense lesion of the pancreatic tail (*arrows*)

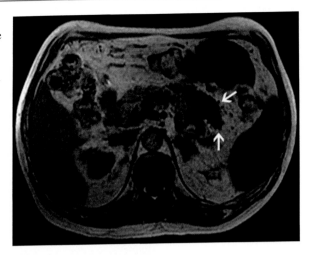

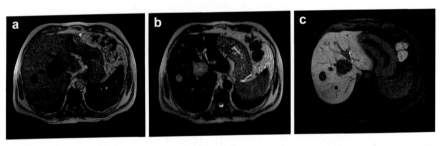

Fig. 4.3 MRI scan: T1w (**a**), T2w, (**b**) and 3D liver acquisition volume acceleration (LAVA sequence) after hepatospecific contrast medium (**c**) show several PNET's liver metastases

4.5   US-CEUS-EUS

US plays a role only in the evaluation of abdominal NET in particular pancreatic tumors (PNET) [6].

Nonfunctional tumors can grow and create a large abdominal mass; in this case US is usually the first imaging technique used for the diagnosis and can guide the transabdominal biopsy.

In the suspicion of functional tumors, which are often small, US has a low sensitivity (ranging from 20 to 86%) [7], which increases with the size of the lesion, while endoscopy with EUS and EUS-FNA has become a cornerstone in the diagnosis of these tumors. Given the limitations also of CT and MRI for small lesions, EUS has become an integral part of the diagnosis of PNETs because of its high sensitivity (from 83 to 94%) [7, 8] in detecting, localizing, and diagnosing pancreatic PNETs.

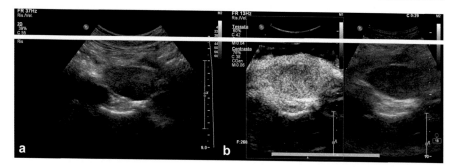

Fig. 4.4 (**a**) Transabdominal ultrasound: hypoechoic, well-defined, homogeneous, pancreatic NET. (**b**) At CEUS the lesion shows enhancement in the arterial phase (29 s after injection of SonoVue)

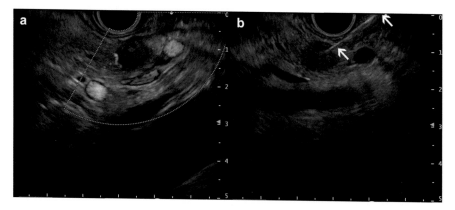

Fig. 4.5 (**a**) EUS: hypoechoic, well-defined, homogeneous, pancreatic NET. (**b**) FNA of the lesion using a 22-gauge needle (*arrows*) (Courtesy of Dr. Pietro Fusaroli, University of Bologna)

Despite EUS and improved radiological imaging, small PNETs may be difficult to localize. Intraoperative palpation combined with intraoperative ultrasound is over 95 % sensitive [9].

Most commonly, PNETs appear hypoechoic, round, homogeneous, and well defined on US (Fig. 4.4a), though they may be isoechoic and, rarely, hyperechoic with irregular margins. Malignant PNETs are larger, with irregular margins, compared to benign PNETs. Classically CEUS, as well as CT and MRI, shows hypervascular enhancement during the arterial phase due to their vascular nature [3] (Fig. 4.4b).

Cystic lesions are the least common presentation, accounting for 8–17 % of PNETs, and may be unilocular, septated, microcystic, or mixed solid-cystic [10].

The addition of FNA to EUS using a 22- or 25-gauge needle enables tissue diagnosis, which allows differentiation from pancreatic adenocarcinoma and is more relevant for diagnosis of nonfunctioning or cystic PNETs (Fig. 4.5).

To improve FNA yield, ideally onsite cytopathology examination should be performed. This examination significantly reduces the rate of unsatisfactory cytology specimens.

> **Key Points**
> - NETs are vascularized tumors in the arterial phase of all contrast imaging techniques.
> - Small PNETs and gastrointestinal NET can be visualized only during EUS or surgical examination.
> - MRI has better diagnostic capabilities in comparison to CT, but it is less available and has several technical limitations.
> - The integration of the different imaging modalities available nowadays allows higher sensitivity and specificity in diagnosing NETs.

References

1. Leung D, Schwartz L. Imaging of neuroendocrine tumors. Semin Oncol. 2013;40:109–19.
2. ENETS guidelines: TNM grading, standard of care and metastasis. www.enets.org.
3. Piscaglia F, et al. The EFSUMB Guidelines and Recommendations on the Clinical Practice of Contrast Enhanced Ultrasound (CEUS): update 2011 on non-hepatic applications. Ultraschall Med. 2011;33:33–59.
4. Sowa-Staszczak A, et al. Are RECIST criteria sufficient to assess response to therapy in neuroendocrine tumors? Clin Imaging. 2012;36(4):360–4.
5. Ramage JK, et al. Guidelines for the management of gastroenteropancreatic neuroendocrine (including carcinoid) tumours (NETs). Gut. 2012;61:6–32.
6. Rockall AG. Imaging of neuroendocrine tumors (CT/MR/US). Best Pract Res Clin Endocrinol Metab. 2007;21(1):43–68.
7. Anderson MA, et al. Endoscopic ultrasound is highly accurate and directs management in patients with neuroendocrine tumors of the pancreas. Am J Gastroenterol. 2000;95:2271–7.
8. Pais SA, et al. EUS for pancreatic neuroendocrine tumors: a single-center, 11-year experience. Gastrointest Endosc. 2010;71:1185–93.
9. Wong M, et al. Intraoperative ultrasound with palpation is still superior to intra-arterial calcium stimulation test in localising insulinoma. World J Surg. 2007;31:586–92.
10. Bordeianou L, et al. Cystic pancreatic endocrine neoplasms: a distinct tumor type? J Am Coll Surg. 2008;206:1154–8.

Radionuclide Imaging (SPECT)

5

Giovanna Pepe and Margarita Kirienko

Contents

5.1   Introduction

Several morphological and functional diagnostic techniques can be used for localizing and assessing the extent of neuroendocrine tumours (NET), but no single imaging technique represents the gold standard, and specific sequences of exams are needed for each tumour type.

Nuclear medicine plays a fundamental role in the study of NETs having the capability to image in vivo the amine pathway and the overexpression of the somatostatin receptors (SSTR), especially SSTR-2, using specific radiopharmaceuticals designed for either scintigraphy or positron emission tomography-computed tomography (PET-CT) [1, 2].

Although the use of PET-CT is increasing, the clinical practice still benefits from the well-established and widely diffused single-photon emission computed tomography (SPECT).

G. Pepe (✉)
Nuclear Medicine, Humanitas Research Hospital, Milan, Italy
e-mail: giovanna.pepe@cancercenter.humanitas.it

M. Kirienko
Nuclear Medicine, Niguarda – Cà Granda Hospital, University Milano Bicocca, Milan, Italy

© Springer International Publishing Switzerland 2016
V. Ambrosini, S. Fanti (eds.), *PET/CT in Neuroendocrine Tumors*,
Clinicians' Guides to Radionuclide Hybrid Imaging: PET/CT,
DOI 10.1007/978-3-319-29203-8_5

Two main groups of radiopharmaceuticals are available:

• Meta-iodo-benzyl-guanidine (mIBG), a norepinephrine analogue that enters the adrenergic pathway
• Somatostatin analogues that bind somatostatin receptors

mIBG is available labelled with ^{131}I or ^{123}I, but nowadays ^{131}I is usually devoted only to therapy applications.

With the introduction of ^{111}In-DTPA-d-Phe1-octreotide, known as ^{111}In-pentetreotide (Octreoscan, Mallinckrodt Medical), that shows the highest affinity for SSTR-2, somatostatin receptor imaging got really started. Other tracers have been developed as the ^{111}In-DOTA-lanreotide (relatively high affinity for SSTR-5, but low affinity for sSSTR2) and those labelled with ^{99m}Tc (^{99m}Tc-EDDA/HYNIC-TOC, ^{99m}Tc-EDDA/HYNIC-TATE, licenced in Eastern Europe).

5.2 Indications to SPECT Imaging

The European Association of Nuclear Medicine (EANM) in the last years gathered its efforts to assist nuclear medicine physicians in the imaging of NETs, with the publication of guidelines for both mIBG scintigraphy and somatostatin receptor scintigraphy (SRS) [3, 4].

Indications are (as summarized in Table 5.1):

• The detection of primary tumours and metastatic sites for staging and restaging purposes (Figs. 5.1, 5.2, and 5.3)
• The assessment of the response to treatment (Fig. 5.4)
• The selection for nuclear medicine therapy

Clinical applications for mIBG are phaeochromocytomas, neuroblastomas, paragangliomas, medullary thyroid carcinoma (MTC) or in multiple endocrine neoplasia (MEN) type 2 syndrome (Table 5.2).

For phaeochromocytomas the overall sensitivity of mIBG imaging reported in literature is 85% and the described specificity is 89%; for neuroblastomas

Table 5.1 Indications to mIBG scintigraphy and SRS

Indication	mIBG	SRS
Detection of primary tumours and of metastatic sites (staging and restaging)	✓	✓
Detect relapse or progression of disease (monitoring patients with known NET)	✓	✓
Predict response to therapy (prognostic evaluation)		✓
Monitor the effects of treatment: surgery, chemo- or radiotherapy	✓	✓
Select patients for mIBG treatment	✓	
Select patients for therapy with radiolabelled peptides		✓

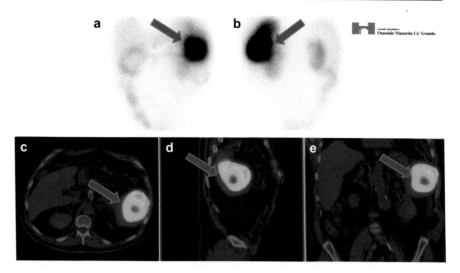

Fig. 5.1 Seventy-six-year-old male referred to Octreoscan for characterization of a pancreatic tale lesion serendipitously detected on CT. Anterior and posterior (**a, b**) planar and SPECT/CT axial, sagittal and coronal (**c–e**) images showed intense uptake of the peripheral part of the lesion (*red arrow*). The patient was scheduled for distal pancreatectomy and splenectomy. In the surgical theatre, intraoperative ultrasound of the liver detected a metastatic lesion, not visualized at preoperative imaging. Pathology characterized the pancreatic lesion as a moderately differentiated pancreatic neuroendocrine tumour (*NET G2 according to WHO classification*) metastatic to the lymph nodes and the liver (pT2 N1 M1)

sensitivity is 92 % and specificity up to 100 % [5, 6]. For MTC the sensitivity is lower, but mIBG can be used to evaluate the relapse of disease after surgery.

SRS is usually requested for the evaluation of gastro-entero-pancreatic (GEP) NETs (e.g. gastrinoma, insulinoma, glucagonoma) and lung carcinoids and less frequently for phaeochromocytoma, neuroblastoma and paraganglioma (Table 5.2).

The sensitivity reported in literature for SRS in GEPs is high, ranging between 70 and 90 % as well as the diagnostic accuracy for primary lesion and metastatic site detection [5].

The sensitivity in lung carcinoids is high for the primary lesion, but lower for the distant metastasis.

The implementation of CT in gamma camera systems was recently shown to improve these results [7]. In a review by Fukuoka et al. [8], CT combination with SPECT was of additional value when compared to scintigraphy alone in 53 % of the studies analysing ^{131}I-mIGB scintigraphy and in 81 % of the studies on ^{123}I-mIBG.

Similar data have been collected for SRS with better sensitivity and specificity when using multimodality imaging instead of scintigraphy or CT alone.

SPECT is mandatory to assess the actual uptake of the radiopharmaceuticals in the lesions in order to select patient candidate to treatment with radiolabelled peptides.

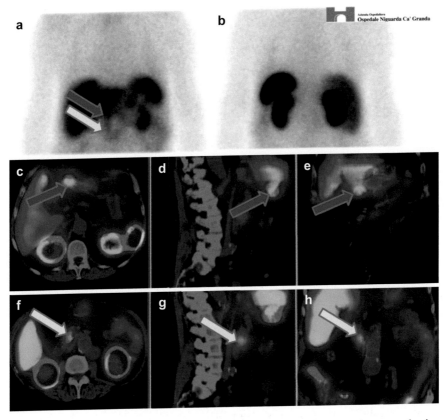

Fig. 5.2 Seventy-nine-year-old male referred to Octreoscan for staging a gastric neuroendocrine tumour. Anterior and posterior (**a**, **b**) planar and SPECT/CT axial, sagittal and coronal (**c–h**) images showed tracer uptake in the pylorus (*red arrows*) and in the duodenum (*yellow arrows*). The lesions turned out to be carcinoids

5.3   Advantages/Limitations/Pitfalls

[123]I/[131]I mIBG traditionally is the first option for radionuclide imaging of phaeo-chromocytomas and neuroblastomas. However, ^{123}I-mIBG compared to ^{131}I-mIBG yields better quality images due to higher resolution. ^{123}I-mIBG adrenal gland normal uptake is lower compared to ^{131}I-mIBG, improving image interpretation.

Whole-body mIBG scan allows the preoperative identification of multiple primary and secondary lesions and, not being affected by postsurgical or post-radiotherapy changes, can detect small recurrences.

False-negative findings could be related to small lesion and/or lesions close to areas of physiological uptake. Lower sensitivity has been reported in paragangliomas, especially in the head and neck region, in familial forms and poorly differentiated malignant tumours.

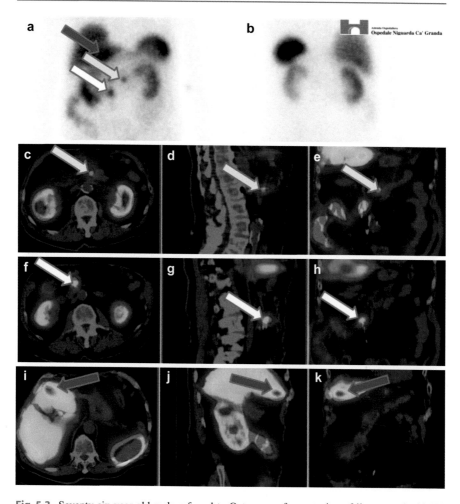

Fig. 5.3 Seventy-six-year-old male referred to Octreoscan for restaging of ileum carcinoid (T3 N1 G1) operated on 4 years earlier. A suspicious mesenteric lymph node was detected on CT. Anterior and posterior planar (**a**, **b**) and SPECT/CT axial, sagittal and coronal (**c–i**, **j**, **k**) images showed tracer uptake at mesenteric lymph nodes (*yellow* and *white arrows*). Furthermore, a liver lesion (*red arrows*) was detected and subsequently confirmed at magnetic resonance imaging with hepato-specific contrast medium

Bilateral adrenal increased uptake, no thyroid blockade and full bladder can mask a pathological uptake. mIBG accumulation within the urinary tract or bowel can be a source of false-positive results.

Some cardiovascular, neurological and sympathomimetic drugs can interfere with the specific mIBG uptake mechanism [5, 9].

SRS is useful for staging, allowing the assessment of liver and extrahepatic metastasis, thus providing important information for therapy decision-making. When positive it has the advantage to predict response to somatostatin analogue treatment.

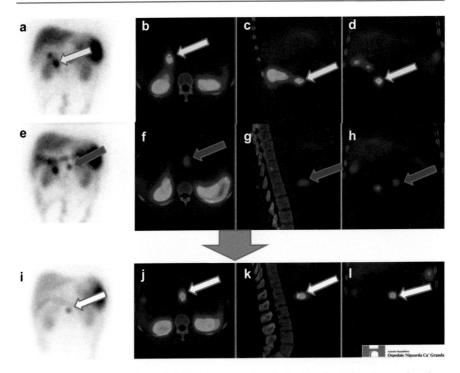

Fig. 5.4 Thirty-five-year-old male affected by MEN1 syndrome; the patient was referred to Octreoscan for staging and lesion characterization, due to Zollinger-Ellison syndrome. Anterior planar (**a**, **e**) and SPECT/CT axial, sagittal and coronal (**b–d** and **f–h**) images revealed a lesion in the duodenum (*yellow arrows*) and peripancreatic lymph node metastasis (*red arrows*) from gastrinoma. The patient underwent duodenum-cefalo-pancreatectomy. Two years later the patient repeated the Octreoscan that showed a new para-aortic lymph node metastasis (*white arrows*) on the anterior planar (**i**) and SPECT/CT axial, sagittal and coronal (**j–l**) images

Table 5.2 Clinical applications for mIBG and SRS		$^{131/123}$I-mIBG	SRS
	GEP-NETs	±	++
	NETs of the lung	–	++
	Phaeochromocytoma, paraganglioma	++	±
	Neuroblastoma	++	–
	Medullary thyroid carcinoma	+	±
	Thymic carcinoids	±	±
	Pituitary	–	±

Modified from Pepe et al. [5]

Major drawbacks are related to the physiological biodistribution: high activity in the liver, spleen and delayed gut activity (biliary excretion). Accessory spleen, gallbladder uptake, urine contamination and nasal uptake (para-physiological change during cold) must be taken into account, as possible sources of misinterpretation. A cause of false-negative results is a lack of SSTR-2 expression in some tumours (i.e. insulinomas, MTC and poorly differentiated lesions). The treatment with somatostatin analogues may reduce the uptake in the tumour and/or reduce the normal liver and spleen uptake. Somatostatin produced by tumour itself could compete with the radiopharmaceutical leading to a lower uptake in the lesions.

When interpreting SRS, non-neoplastic diseases such as autoimmune disorders, post-radiation inflammatory disease, granulomatous disease and some bacterial infections should be considered for differential diagnosis [10].

Key Points

- Neuroendocrine tumours (NETs) are heterogeneous albeit sharing some metabolic features that are useful targets for functional imaging with high sensitivity and specificity.
- The catecholamine pathway can be imaged using mIBG, a norepinephrine analogue.
- The expression of somatostatin receptors can be in vivo investigated using radiolabelled somatostatin analogues.
- Clinical applications for mIBG are phaeochromocytomas, neuroblastomas, paragangliomas, MTC alone or in MEN2 syndrome.
- Somatostatin receptor scintigraphy plays a role in the evaluation of GEP-NETs (gastrinoma, insulinoma, glucagonoma) and lung carcinoids.
- Scintigraphic imaging is still a front-line technique in the diagnostic work-up of NET patients: it is well established worldwide and procedural guidelines are available.
- Good accuracy is reported for both mIBG and SRS.
- Major drawbacks are related to normal biodistribution and small lesions.
- Scintigraphy is mandatory before selecting patients that can benefit from treatment with iodine-131-labelled mIBG and radiolabelled somatostatin analogues.

References

1. Wong KK, Waterfield RT, Marzola MC, et al. Contemporary nuclear medicine imaging of neuroendocrine tumours. Clin Radiol. 2012;67:1035–50.
2. van Essen M, Sundin A, Krenning EP, et al. Neuroendocrine tumours: the role of imaging for diagnosis and therapy. Nat Rev Endocrinol. 2014;10:102–14. doi:10.1038/nrendo.2013.246.
3. Bombardieri E, Giammarile F, Aktolun C, et al. 131I/123I Metaiodobenzylguanidine (mIBG) scintigraphy: procedure guidelines for tumour imaging. Eur J Nucl Med Mol Imaging. 2010;37:2436–46.
4. Bombardieri E, Ambrosini V, Aktolun C, et al. 111In-pentetreotide scintigraphy: procedure guidelines for tumour imaging. Eur J Nucl Med Mol Imaging. 2010;37:1441–8.
5. Pepe G, Bombardieri E, Lorenzoni A, Chiti A. Single-photon emission computed tomography tracers in the diagnostics of neuroendocrine tumors. PET Clin. 2014;9(1):11–26.
6. Ilias I, Chen CC, Carrasquillo JA, et al. Comparison of 6-(18) F-fluorodopamine PET with I-123-metaiodobenzylguanidine and in-111-pentetreotide scintigraphy in localization of non-metastatic and metastatic pheochromocytoma. J Nucl Med. 2008;49:1613–9.

7. Fuccio C, Spinapolice EG, Chondrogiannis S, et al. Evolving role of SPECT/CT in neuroendocrine tumors management staging, treatment response, and follow-up. Clin Nucl Med. 2013;38(10):e384–9.
8. Fukuoka M, Taki J, Mochizuki T, et al. Comparison of diagnostic value of I-123 MIBG and high dose I-131 MIBG scintigraphy including incremental value of SPECT/CT over planar image in patients with malignant pheochromocytoma/paraganglioma and neuroblastoma. Clin Nucl Med. 2011;36:1–7.
9. Volterrani D, Orsini F, Chiacchio S, Bodei L. Multiagent targeting of neuroendocrine neoplasms. Clin Transl Imaging. 2013;1:407–21. doi:10.1007/s40336-013-0043-x.
10. Toumpanakis C, Kim MK, Rinke A, et al. Combination of cross-sectional and molecular imaging studies in the localization of gastroenteropancreatic neuroendocrine tumors. Neuroendocrinology. 2014;99:63–74. doi:10.1159/000358727. Advanced Release: January 21, 2014.

Basic Principles of PET-CT Imaging

6

Deborah Tout, John Dickson, and Andy Bradley

Contents

6.1 Introduction

PET-CT imaging has become a very powerful tool in cancer imaging; it utilises the detection of the radiation emitted from radionuclides that decay by positron (β^+) emission. This chapter looks into the physical principles of this technique, factors that affect the quality of the images produced and some of the artefacts and problems that may be encountered.

D. Tout (✉)
Biomedical Technology Services, Gold Coast University Hospital, Southport, QLD, Australia
e-mail: Deborah.Tout@health.qld.gov.uk

J. Dickson
Nuclear Medicine Department, University College London Hospitals NHS Foundation Trust, London, UK

A. Bradley
Nuclear Medicine Centre, Manchester Royal Infirmary, Manchester, UK

© Springer International Publishing Switzerland 2016
V. Ambrosini, S. Fanti (eds.), *PET/CT in Neuroendocrine Tumors*,
Clinicians' Guides to Radionuclide Hybrid Imaging: PET/CT,
DOI 10.1007/978-3-319-29203-8_6

6.2   Positron Emission Tomography (PET)

Positron emission tomography (PET) is the imaging of radiopharmaceuticals labelled with positron-emitting radionuclides. Positrons are the positively charged antimatter version of the electron and are ejected during the radioactive decay of a proton-rich nucleus; during this decay process, a proton in the nucleus is converted into a neutron. The positron is ejected from the nucleus carrying a lot of kinetic energy; it then travels a short distance and undergoes a number of interactions with the surrounding atoms. In each interaction the positron loses some kinetic energy and changes its direction of travel, following a random path through the surrounding matter. When the positron is at rest, it annihilates with a nearby electron. Due to the conservation of energy, the energy associated with their combined mass (rest mass energy; $E=mc^2$) is converted to two annihilation photons each with energy of 511 keV. Conservation of momentum dictates that the two photons are emitted from the point of annihilation travelling in opposite directions (Fig. 6.1). These properties, the instantaneous production of two photons of equal energy travelling 180 degrees to each other, are the basis of the PET imaging technique used to localise where the original annihilation event occured within the patient.

A PET scanner is composed of several rings of small crystal scintillation detectors. Each detector is a few mm in size, and a group of them are formed into a block that is typically connected to a group of four photomultiplier tubes. The scintillator detectors convert incoming photons into light before amplifying the signal using the photomultiplier tubes. When there is a positron emission within the ring of detectors, the two 511 keV photons, travelling at the speed of light, will be detected almost instantaneously (within approximately 10 ns). Photons arriving at different detectors within this coincidence timing window are called coincidence events. The

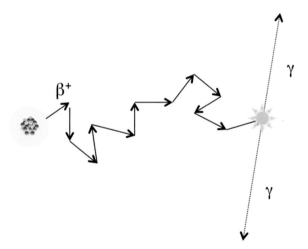

Fig. 6.1 During a nuclear decay, a positron is emitted from a nucleus and undergoes a series of interactions with atoms in the surrounding tissue. When its kinetic energy is almost zero, it and a neighbouring electron annihilate turning the mass of the two particles into energy in the form of two 511 keV photons. (Nucleus and random walk are not to scale)

line between the two detectors that detected each coincidence event is called the 'line of response'. Typically data are collected over several minutes and all detected coincidence events are grouped into parallel lines of response to form projections through the patient that are used for image reconstruction, typically using iterative reconstruction techniques. The great advantage of this type of localisation is that, unlike a gamma camera, it does not require collimators to provide positional information and therefore offers much higher sensitivity than single-photon emission computed tomography (SPECT).

The type of coincidence event described above is called a 'true' coincidence, and it is these signals that create the useful image. There are however other unwanted coincidence events that can occur (Fig. 6.2). A 'random' coincidence event is where multiple positron emissions and annihilations occurring in quick succession lead to a number of photons arriving at the detectors within the coincidence time window. If the wrong pair of detected photons is seen as the coincidence event, this will lead to an incorrect line of response. This process is called a random event as the line of response is not associated with a true annihilation event. The proportion of random events to total coincidence events increases significantly with higher activity concentrations and larger coincidence acceptance time windows, e.g. by moving from 10 to 15 ns. A 'scattered' event is where one or both photons coming from a positron-electron annihilation are scattered during their path to the detectors; the line of response will again be incorrect. The fraction of coincidence events that can be attributed to scatter increases with increased scattering material i.e. larger or denser tissue. Although unwanted coincidences can degrade image quality, all modern image reconstruction techniques use correction algorithms, which limit the effect of these types of event.

Along with adjustments for scattered and random events, there are other corrections that need to be applied during the reconstruction process to increase the accuracy of the final image. These include dead time corrections to deal with the high count rates found in PET and a normalisation correction to correct for the difference in measured signal across pairs of detectors used to give the lines of response. However, the most dramatic of the corrections applied in PET is that to correct for photon attenuation within the patient. Although the photons in PET are more energetic than those in single-photon tomography, both photons need to be detected for a

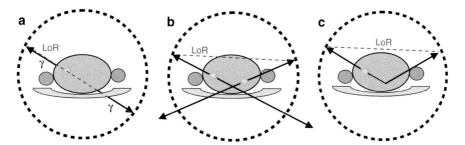

Fig. 6.2 Coincidence events in PET. (**a**) A true event with correct line of response (*LoR*), (**b**) a random event with two unrelated annihilations registering an incorrect line of response, (**c**) a scattered event where one photon has been scattered leading to an incorrectly positioned line of response

signal to be registered; this means that the full thickness of patient tissue traversed by both photons affects the relative attenuation of signal from different parts of the patient. The effects of photon attenuation are therefore more dramatic in PET than in SPECT and lead to the classic 'hot' skin and lungs on uncorrected images (Fig. 6.3).

Exact attenuation correction (AC) is relatively straightforward so long as an accurate attenuation map is known. With the advent of PET-CT, the CT scan, which effectively is a map of attenuation at X-ray energies, can, with appropriate conversion factors, provide attenuation correction maps in a matter of seconds. The CT is mounted in the same gantry as the PET, and the bed moves the patient between the two scanners for sequential imaging. There are issues to be considered when using attenuation maps derived from CT, such as accurate translation of attenuation coefficients from lower-energy X-ray photons to 511 keV; potential misregistration due to patient and respiratory motion; the use of contrast agents leading to incorrect attenuation maps owing to their enhanced attenuation only at the lower X-ray energies; and the presence of metal artefacts and the additional radiation dose to the patient. Despite these limitations, the use of CT for AC has grown rapidly because of the low statistical noise in the attenuation maps and the addition of registered anatomical information; the fusion of CT with PET greatly enhances the interpretation of the functional information as will be seen through most of this book.

More recent technical advances include resolution (point-spread-function) modelling in PET image reconstruction resulting in significant improvements in image resolution and contrast. Also modern fast crystal detectors are able to more precisely record the difference in the arrival times of the coincidence photons, known as time-of-flight (TOF) imaging. TOF helps localise the point of origin of the annihilation event along the line of response. The reduction in noise offered by TOF can be equated to a gain in sensitivity.

An advantage of applying a comprehensive set of corrections in PET-CT is that, with the inclusion of a sensitivity calibration, there is the possibility to calculate voxel values in terms of activity concentration per unit volume (kBq/ml). This activity concentration will change with patient size or administered activity so it becomes

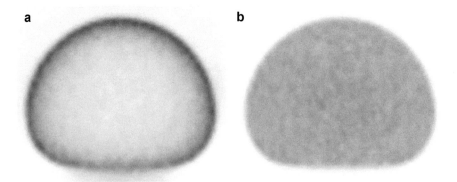

Fig. 6.3 Images of a trans-axial slice through a phantom filled with a uniform solution of fluorine-18 (**a**) without correction for photon attenuation and (**b**) with attenuation correction

more useful if this uptake is represented as a value normalised by the available activity concentration in the body. This is achieved by normalising for injected activity and body size (weight or lean body mass), and this leads to the semiquantitative index known as standardised uptake values (SUV). The SUV in each voxel will equal 1 for a uniform distribution. SUV is defined as

$$SUV(g/ml) = \frac{Activity\,concentration\,(kBq/ml)}{Administered\,activity\,(MBq)/\,Weight\,(kg)}$$

SUV was defined for use in PET whole body oncology imaging with fluorine-18-fluorodeoxyglucose (usually abbreviated as [18F]FDG or just FDG). Most PET display workstations will display PET images in SUV. Although the use of SUV is widespread, there are many factors that can affect its accuracy. It requires accurate measurement of administered activity, injection time, scan time and patient weight and is affected by the performance characteristics of the PET scanner and image reconstruction factors. SUV also has a strong positive correlation with body weight. Heavy patients have a higher percentage of body fat that contributes to body weight but accumulates little FDG in the fasting state, so SUVs in non-fatty tissues are increased in larger patients. SUV normalised to lean body mass or body surface area has been shown to have a lesser dependence on body weight, although SUV normalised to body weight is still the most clinically used parameter. Many physiological factors can affect SUV, including scan delay time (accumulation of FDG continues to increase over time), patient resting state, temperature, blood glucose level, insulin levels and renal clearance. In addition FDG is not a specific tumour marker, and uptake will be high in areas affected by infective or inflammatory processes that are often seen immediately post-chemotherapy.

Several values of SUV can be quoted, the most common being SUV_{max} which is robust and relatively independent of the observer, but as it refers to a single voxel value, it is strongly affected by image noise and can change significantly depending on count statistics and reconstruction parameters. It may also not be representative of the overall uptake in a heterogeneous tumour. SUV_{mean} is more representative of the average tumour uptake and is less affected by image noise, but can be prone to observer variability if freely drawn regions are used. Although the SUV formula has been criticised, the simplicity of the calculation makes it extremely attractive for routine clinical use.

There is a wide range of positron-emitting radionuclides used in PET (Table 6.1). Many have a short half-life, which requires an expensive cyclotron production facility on the same site as the PET-CT scanner. Fluorine-18 has a slightly longer half-life allowing it to be transported from the production facility to other imaging sites. This explains the popularity of fluorinated PET radiopharmaceuticals such as FDG. There are also longer half-life radionuclides such as copper-64 which allows imaging of pharmaceuticals with slower uptake kinetics. However, not all PET radionuclides require a cyclotron. Generators also exist, similar to the molybdenum-99/technetium-99m generator, which can produce PET radionuclides repeatedly on site. Gallium-68 and rubidium-82 are popular, short-lived, generator-produced PET radionuclides; gallium-68 comes from germanium-68 parent and rubidium-82 from strontium-82 parent.

Table 6.1 Properties of some radionuclides used in clinical PET imaging [1, 2]

Radionuclide	Half-life (min)	Average range (mm)	Positron fraction	Generator produced
Carbon-11	20.4	1.1	100	No
Nitrogen-13	9.96	1.5	100	No
Oxygen-15	2.03	2.5	100	No
Fluorine-18	110	0.6	97	No
Copper-64	762	0.6	18	No
Gallium-68	68	2.9	88	Yes
Rubidium-82	1.25	5.9	95	Yes

Not all radioactive decays result in the emission of a positron; for example, with copper-64, only 18 % of decays produce positrons. This means that the sensitivity of the PET scanner to copper-64 labelled compounds is less than a fifth of that possible with fluorine-18. There may also be additional radiations resulting from the other decay routes or contaminants which can affect patient and staff radiation exposure and image quality.

The average range of the positron is important as it determines the distance the positron travels before the creation of the annihilation photons; this range is dependent on the initial energy of the positron following the radioactive decay. Because the positron moves through tissue in a random path, it is not possible to know the exact point in the tissue where the original decay took place. Spatial resolution in the images depends, to some extent, on the average range of the positron in that tissue. As a result, the spatial resolution of gallium-68 and rubidium-82 imaging will be worse than that from fluorine-18 tracers. The average positron ranges given in Table 6.1 are for soft tissue; the range of a positron will be much greater in air.

By far the most common radiopharmaceutical currently used in PET imaging is [F-18]FDG. Although FDG is a glucose analogue, it does not enter the glycolytic pathway after phosphorylation, but becomes trapped in the cell allowing imaging of FDG concentration, which infers glycolytic rate. Both glucose and FDG are filtered by the glomeruli, but unlike glucose, FDG is not reabsorbed by tubuli and therefore appears in urine. [F-18]FDG PET has become an important tool in oncology imaging for diagnosis and staging and to evaluate metabolic changes in tumours at the cellular level. Although very sensitive for imaging many cancer types, it is also non-specific, detecting many other physiological processes such as inflammation and infection.

6.3   PET Scanning

PET-CT imaging usually starts with a localising scan projection radiograph often known as a 'scout' or 'topogram' where the extent of PET scanning is defined. The patient then has a CT scan of this defined length that will be used for attenuation correction and possibly uptake localisation, before moving through the scanner bore for the PET scan. The axial PET field of view which defines the amount of body that can be scanned in one stop is normally around 15 cm, although systems are now available that scan 22 cm or even 26 cm. For brain scanning or cardiac scanning, only one field of view is required; however in oncology imaging where the extent of disease is often of interest, whole-body imaging can be performed. This is typically done by acquiring several fields of view with a slight overlap to allow for the detector sensitivity losses at the edges of the field of view (Fig. 6.4). Each of these fields of view is called a bed position, and the time of each scan at these bed positions can be between 1.5 and 5 min in duration, depending on the affinity of the radiopharmaceutical and the sensitivity of the scanner. Patients should be made comfortable and immobilised when necessary to keep the patient in the same position to maintain registration between the PET and the CT used for attenuation correction and localisation and limit movement artefacts.

For some applications, dynamic PET imaging over a single bed position can be useful to understand patient physiology. However, it is more typical to start PET imaging after a fixed period of time; this uptake or resting time is determined by the physiological uptake and excretion of the administered tracer with the aim to scan at the optimum time to have a good uptake in the target tissue with a low

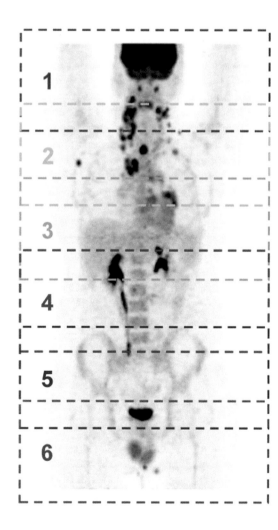

Fig. 6.4 A whole body image is made up of multiple bed positions that are stitched together; in this example six acquisitions are required to cover the desired length of the patient

background circulation of the tracer in the rest of the body. For repeat imaging to assess disease progression, it is important to keep this uptake time duration similar for successive imaging, typically within ±5 min.

6.4   Imaging with [Fluorine-18]FDG PET

The patient must arrive well hydrated and have fasted for between 4 and 6 h to ensure blood glucose levels are low prior to injection with FDG. This is to ensure that there is limited competition between FDG and existing blood glucose, so that uptake of FDG is maximised in order to give the best possible image quality. Care needs to be taken with diabetic patients. A patient history should be taken to determine when the patient last had radiotherapy or chemotherapy. FDG uptake can be elevated as a reactive response to these treatments. It is also important to remember that FDG can be sensitive to inflammation/infection, so a general understanding of the patients' wellbeing and history of recent physical trauma (including biopsy) is necessary. For SUV calculations, patients' weight (and height if correcting for lean body mass) should be taken with reliable calibrated instruments to ensure accurate quantification of uptake. Injection of FDG should be intravenous through an indwelling cannula and the clocks used to record the injection and scan times should be calibrated; any discrepancies in the recorded times can lead to errors in the decay correction used for quantification of the uptake. All PET tracers are beta emitters (a beta particle is a high energy electron or positron), so particular care should be taken to reduce the likelihood of extravasation and local radiation burden. To assist in the quantification of FDG uptake, the exact injected activity of FDG should be recorded.

Imaging typically starts at 60 min postinjection, and the patients must rest and be kept warm during this uptake period to avoid unwanted muscle or brown fat uptake. Patients are asked to void prior to imaging to reduce the activity in the bladder; full bladders containing high activity of FDG can cause difficulties in interpreting the images around this region and also increases the radiation dose to staff while the patient is positioned on the scanner bed. A multiple bed-position whole-body scan is normally performed from the mid-thigh up to the base of the brain. FDG is processed via renal excretion, so it is important where possible to scan in this direction to avoid scanning a bladder that has refilled with FDG during the scan. With the patient lying supine, whole body imaging is performed with the arms raised above the patient's head to avoid CT beam hardening artefacts and to ensure that the patient's body fits within the trans-axial field of view. If head and neck imaging is required, an additional arms down scan over the head and neck area can be helpful to reduce attenuation in this area.

6.5   Artefacts

There are several artefacts that can occur in PET imaging even when all reasonable precautions are taken. One of the hardest artefacts to control is due to respiratory motion that can occur if the patient takes a large breath hold prior to or during the

CT. As can be seen in Fig. 6.5a, the result can be a banana-shaped artefact caused by mismatch of PET and CT used for attenuation correction at the base of the lung and dome of the liver. The easiest way to avoid these artefacts is to ensure that the patient is relaxed prior to imaging and ask them not to take any large intakes of breath – particularly during the CT. Other motion-related artefacts are standard patient movement such as that seen in Fig. 6.5b. Relatively common in head and neck imaging, the mismatch of CT and PET can lead to incorrect attenuation correction and difficulty in localising features. Making the patient feel relaxed, helping them understand the need to remain still and appropriate immobilisation can help reduce the likelihood of these artefacts.

An artefact that cannot be easily controlled is the CT X-ray beam hardening, and subsequent streaking aretefacts in the CT image, produced by metal prosthesis typically in the hip or where the patient has metal dental work (Fig. 6.6). Many modern systems have algorithms that can help minimise these effects. Nevertheless, care must be taken when quantifying uptake in affected areas because inaccuracies in the attenuation map derrived from the CT data can lead to inaccuracies in PET quantification. Another area where attenuation correction can fail is when CT contrast has been used. The conversion of the attenuation map derived from CT X-ray energies to attenuation values at PET photon energies can fail in areas of CT contrast accumulation. This is due to the elevated attenuation of contrast media, such as iodine and barium, at the lower X-ray energies due to the K-edge absorption peak; this peak does not affect the absorption of the 511 keV PET photons. As the reconstruction algorithm cannot distinguish between tissue that has a high density and less

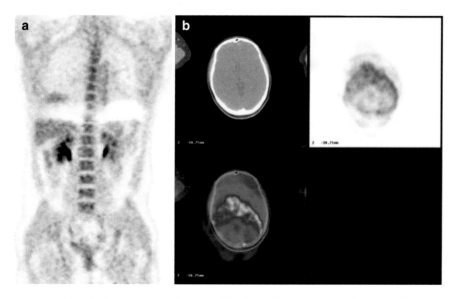

Fig. 6.5 (**a**) Respiratory motion artefact seen at the dome of the liver caused by mismatch of PET and CT for attenuation correction. (**b**) Patient motion between CT for attenuation correction and PET leading to poor correction for attenuation and localisation of tracer uptake

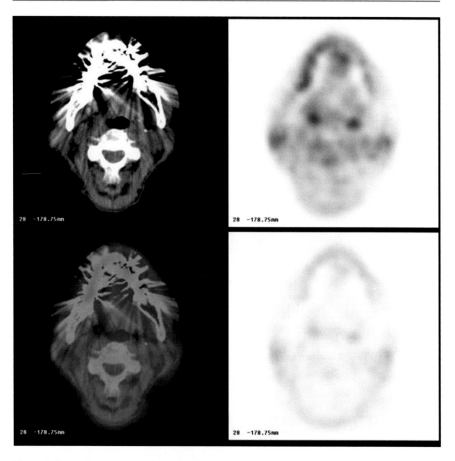

Fig. 6.6 Beam hardening artefacts on CT caused by dental amalgam. PET quantification and localisation can be difficult although non-attenuation-corrected data (*bottom right panel*) may help with identifying artefacts in the attenuation-corrected images (*top right panel*)

dense tissue containing CT contrast, the attenuation correction overcorrects areas containing contrast. This again can lead to errors in PET quantification. If quantification is particularly important, e.g. in a trial setting, the contrast CT should be performed last after the PET data is acquired, and the attenuation correction should be performed using a low-dose CT acquired before the contrast administration.

An important tool to identiy many artefacts introduced during the attenuation correction process is the reading of PET images without attenuation correction. Although these images are then not quantitative, they can be useful to highlight areas of artefact and to assess disease within the patient.

Careful consideration of radiation protection is important due to the high-energy annihilation photons. Over ten times the thickness of lead is required to shield PET photons compared to 140 keV photons, and, immediately post injection, the dose rate from a patient administered with fluorine-18 is ten times that of a patient administered with the same activity of technetium-99m. Extremity dose to staff can be high when handling PET tracers due to the positron radiations.

The short physical half-lives of PET tracers result in a lower patient dose than might be expected. A typical administered activity of 350 MBq [F-18]FDG corresponds to an effective dose of approximately 7 mSv, and with ongoing improvements in PET detector technology and reconstruction methods, both imaging times and typical administered activities are decreasing. The required level of CT image quality (and therefore effective dose) depends on the use of the CT data. When the CT data are used solely for AC, patient doses can be extremely low (<1 mSv). A notable improvement in image quality (and dose increase) is required if the CT data are to be used for AC and anatomical localization (typically 3–8 mSv), and a further increase in both image quality and dose is required if the CT images are to be used for diagnostic purposes, usually with the addition of contrast agents (typically >15 mSv).

Key Points
- Positron emission tomography (PET) is the imaging of radiopharmaceuticals labelled with positron-emitting radionuclides.
- Positron decay leads to two 511 keV photons following annihilation of the emitted positron and a nearby electron.
- $E = mc^2$. Positron mass $= 9.109 \times 10^{-31}$ g, speed of light $= 2.9979 \times 10^8$ m/s and 1 eV $= 1.6 \times 10^{-19}$ J. You know you want to do the calculation.
- A PET scanner is composed of several rings of scintillation detectors.
- Coincident detection of the two photons in different detectors allows an image to be formed from information gleaned by tracking 'lines of response' between these detectors.
- TOF helps localise the point of origin of the annihilation event along the line of response. This helps to decrease noise, and thereby improve signal to noise ratio.
- The sensitivity of the scanner drops towards the edges of the axial field of view of the detectors. Adjacent bed positions need to be overlapped to account for this
- A semi-quantitative index, standardised uptake value (SUV) is commonly used in clinical PET.
- Several values of SUV can be quoted, the most common being SUV_{max} which is relatively robust, as it is less affected by the observer than SUV_{mean}, but it is strongly affected by image noise.
- SUV_{mean} is more representative of the average tumour uptake and is less affected by image noise, but can be prone to observer variability.
- To assist in the quantification of FDG uptake, the exact injected activity of FDG should be recorded.
- For SUV calculations, patients' weight (and height if correcting by lean body mass) should be taken with reliable calibrated instruments to ensure accurate quantification of uptake.

- SUV values are affected by changes in reconstruction techniques and can vary between scanners; it is only semi-quantitative.
- Careful patient preparation is important to obtain good-quality PET images.
- All PET tracers are beta emitters, so particular care should be taken to reduce the likelihood of extravasation and local radiation burden.
- There are several artefacts that can occur in PET imaging even when all reasonable precautions are taken; knowledge of these is important when interpreting images.
- The effects of photon attenuation are more dramatic in PET, and attenuation correction is essential.
- A typical administered activity of 350 MBq F-18 FDG corresponds to an effective dose of approximately 7 mSv.
- Radiation doses to staff are much higher when exposed to PET tracers than from similar activities of other technetium-based nuclear medicine tracers.

References

1. NUDAT 2.6, National Nuclear Data Centre, Brookhaven National Laboratory, http://www.nndc.bnl.gov/nudat2/.
2. Cal-Gonzalez J, et al. Positron range effects in high resolution 3D PET imaging. Nuclear science symposium conference record (NSS/MIC), 2009 IEEE Orlando, FL.

PET/CT in Neuroendocrine Tumours

Valentina Ambrosini and Stefano Fanti

Contents

7.1 Introduction

The past three decades have witnessed a radical change in the diagnostic approach to neuroendocrine tumours (NEN). In the early 1990s, Krenning et al. [1] documented the higher diagnostic accuracy of somatostatin receptor scintigraphy (SRS) over conventional morphological procedures (US, CT) for both the detection of the primary tumour and distant metastasis (overall detection rate ranging between 80 and 100 %). In fact the variable presentation of NEN, in terms of both size and

V. Ambrosini, MD, PhD (✉) • S. Fanti, MD
Nuclear Medicine, University of Bologna, S.Orsola-Malpighi Hospital, Bologna, Italy
e-mail: valentina.ambrosini@unibo.it; stefano.fanti@aosp.bo.it

© Springer International Publishing Switzerland 2016
V. Ambrosini, S. Fanti (eds.), *PET/CT in Neuroendocrine Tumors*,
Clinicians' Guides to Radionuclide Hybrid Imaging: PET/CT,
DOI 10.1007/978-3-319-29203-8_7

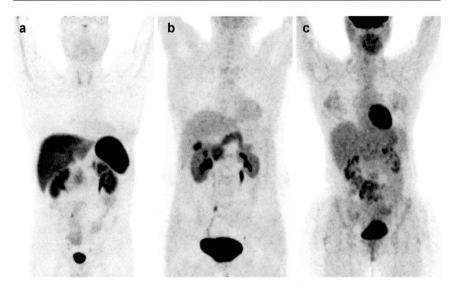

Fig. 7.1 Physiological biodistribution of clinically employed beta-emitting tracers for the assessment of neuroendocrine tumours: (**a**) 68Ga-DOTA-NOC, (**b**)18F-DOPA, and (**c**)18F-FDG

primary tumour site, mainly accounts for the lower performance of conventional imaging modalities. The availability of radiotracers specifically binding to somatostatin receptors (SSTR) overexpressed on NEN cells has represented a major advance in the diagnosis of these tumour forms.

Of course, with the advent of PET/CT, several new beta-emitting tracers have been employed in the clinic with good results, and the role of scintigraphy will become more and more marginal. PET/CT offers several advantages over SRS including a higher spatial resolution and higher accuracy in lesion detection [2], the possibility to semi-quantify the tracer uptake in the region of interest (SUV$_{max}$), lower costs [3] and shorter image acquisition protocol (2 h vs acquisitions at 4–24 h). A recent paper comparing PET/CT with 68Ga-DOTA-TATE (characterised by a high-binding affinity for SSTR-2) with SRS, reported that in patients with negative or weakly positive findings on SRS, PET/CT documented 168 vs 28 lesions [2].

At present, both receptor-based (68Ga-DOTA-peptides) and metabolic (18F-FDG and 18F-DOPA) beta-emitting tracers are available for imaging NEN with PET/CT (Fig. 7.1).

7.2   PET/CT Radiopharmaceuticals and Their Clinical Indications

7.2.1   68Ga-DOTA-Peptides

Currently the most promising tracers to study well-differentiated NEN are represented by a group of beta-emitting radiopharmaceuticals (68Ga-DOTA-peptides) specifically binding to SSTR overexpressed on NEN cells [4, 5].

68Ga-DOTA-peptides present a common structure: a beta-emitting isotope (68Ga), a chelant (DOTA) and the ligand to SSTR (NOC, TOC, TATE). The different clinically employed compounds (68Ga-DOTA-TOC, 68Ga-DOTA-NOC, 68Ga-DOTA-TATE) differ for the binding affinity for SSTR subtypes, with DOTA-TATE presenting the higher affinity for SSTR-2 (the most common receptor on NEN) and DOTA-NOC presenting the wider subtype affinity (binding to SSTR-2, SSTR-3, SSTR-5). At present, these compounds are considered to provide substantially equal information from a clinical point of view: few papers directly comparing one tracer over the other in the same patient group reported comparable diagnostic accuracy. However, it should be reminded that no direct comparison of the SUV_{max} value measured using different compounds can be performed.

68Ga-DOTA-peptides accuracy in NEN lesion detection (Figs. 7.2 and 7.3) is superior to SRS, morphologic imaging procedures and PET/CT with metabolic tracers (18F-FDG, 18F-DOPA).

The synthesis and labelling process of 68Ga-DOTA-peptides is quite easy and economic: gallium can be easily eluted from a commercially available Ge-68/Ga-68 generator, and therefore, there is no need of an on-site cyclotron. 68Gallium ($t_{1/2} = 68$ min) presents an 89% positron emission and negligible gamma emission (1077 keV) of 3.2%. The long half-life of the mother radionuclide 68Ge (270.8 days) makes it possible to use the generator for approximately 9–12 months, depending upon the requirement, rendering the whole procedure relatively economic.

Several papers in the past 5 years reported the high accuracy of these compounds (sensitivity 90–98%, specificity 92–98%) [4, 5] for the detection of NEN in patients studied for staging and restaging after therapy and detection of the unknown primary tumour in cases presenting with metastatic NEN lesions. One indication for 68Ga-DOTA-peptides PET/CT is certainly the possibility to non-invasively assess the presence of SSTR on target cells, therefore representing an unavoidable procedure before starting target therapy with either cold or hot somatostatin analogues (PRRT). 68Ga-DOTA-peptides PET/CT has been reported to provide prognostic information (patients presenting lower SUV_{max} values were more likely to present disease progression) and to have an impact on patient management [6]. Since 68Ga-DOTA-peptides PET/CT uptake correlates with SSTR expression on NET cells, it also provides an indirect measure of cell differentiation: lesions with a high 68Ga-DOTA-peptide uptake have a higher differentiation grade and are therefore associated with a better prognosis and are more likely to respond to treatment with either hot or cold somatostatin analogues (PRRT).

The employment of 68Ga-DOTA-peptides PET/CT as first-step examination in patient with only a clinical suspicion of NEN and the assessment of the response to therapy are on the contrary two clinical settings in which there is debate on whether DOTA-peptides should be routinely employed.

In 2011 [7], the EANM published guidelines for the standardisation of 68Ga-DOTA-peptides PET/CT acquisition, in particular no specific patient preparation is required, and the use of contrast media is not routinely recommended.

Specific metabolic tracers are more suitable than 68Ga-DOTA-peptides for the assessment of tumours presenting with variable to low expression of SSTR (e.g.

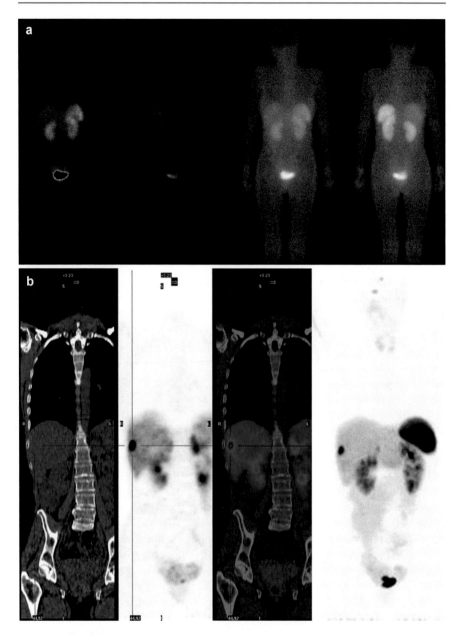

Fig. 7.2   68Ga-DOTA-NOC PET/CT images of a 51-year-old female patient studied for restaging of a well-differentiated neuroendocrine tumour of the pancreas. The patient lamented the onset of pyrosis and diarrhoea to her primary care physician 9 months after surgical excision of the primary tumour. CT detected the presence of a focal lesion at the 8th segment (lesion dimensions, 1.5 × 1.8 cm). SRS was negative, (**a**) while 68Ga-DOTA-NOC PET/CT (**b**) demonstrated a focal area of increased tracer uptake

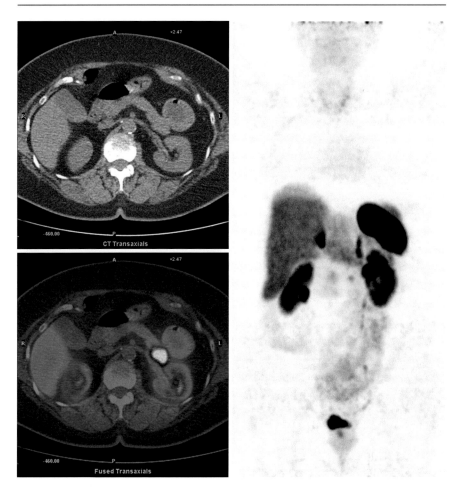

Fig. 7.3 68Ga-DOTA-NOC PET/CT images of a 60-year-old female patient presenting an area of focal uptake at pancreatic tail level ($SUV_{max} = 38$) and local lymph node ($SUV_{max} = 4.6$). Pathology confirmed the neuroendocrine nature of the lesion

undifferentiated forms, neuroblastoma, medullary thyroid cancer, benign insulinoma, pheochromocytoma) or of undifferentiated forms.

7.2.2   18F-DOPA

18F-DOPA is a metabolic tracer that can be successfully employed to study NEN patients. NEN cells belong to the APUD cells system and have therefore the capability to take up, accumulate and decarboxylate amine precursors such as dihydroxyphenylalanine (DOPA) and hydroxytryptophan. Several authors reported good diagnostic accuracy for the detection of NEN lesions and superior sensitivity and specificity as compared to morphological imaging [8].

Studies of direct comparison between 68Ga-DOTA-peptides imaging and 18F-DOPA are few and demonstrate the superiority of 68Ga-DOTA-peptides in well-differentiated forms of NET, for both the detection of the primary tumour and of secondary lesions [5]. These findings, in addition to 68Ga-DOTA-peptides' easy and economic synthesis process and the possibility to study SSTR expression prior to treatment, account for the increasing employment of these compounds over 18F-DOPA in well-differentiated NET.

In fact, the major limit for the widespread use of 18F-DOPA in clinical practice has been represented by the complex and costly synthesis process.

Therefore, the 18F-DOPA main clinical employment is in NEN forms with variable to low expression of SSTR that cannot be accurately studied by 68Ga-DOTA-peptides PET/CT. Currently, 18F-DOPA is successfully employed for imaging neuroblastoma, pheochromocytoma and medullary thyroid carcinoma.

Being a metabolic tracer, another potential clinical setting in which 18F-DOPA may provide additional value is the assessment of the response to therapy.

7.2.3   18F-FDG

Although generally slow growing and presenting with a low glucose metabolic rate, NEN may also show a high proliferation index (ki67) and lower differentiation grade. These forms are more likely to be detected by 18F-FDG [9], and the presence of FDG-positive lesions is associated with a worst outcome. Dual tracer imaging (using both 18F-FDG and 68Ga-DOTA-peptides) has been proposed but is not routinely used and performed only in selected cases.

7.2.4   Practical Consideration on the Choice of the Most Suitable First-Line Tracer for NEN Imaging

Since NEN do not constitute a metabolically and biologically homogenous tumour group, the choice of the most suitable PET/CT tracer should be established on a patient basis and, obviously, tracer availability. Although there is no definitive knowledge in this field and the published data are not sufficient to derive a unique gold standard, the currently used major parameter to address the patient to PET/CT imaging is represented by the 2010 WHO grade classification. Patients with G1 are generally studied with 68Ga-DOTA-peptides, G2 cases are preferentially studied with 68Ga-DOTA-peptides (although for higher ki67 levels or in cases presenting also with SSTR-negative lesions on low-dose CT images FDG may also provide relevant prognostic data) and G3 patients may be studied as first-step examination with 18F-FDG. 18F-DOPA is suitable for well-differentiated tumours (although with lower accuracy than 68Ga-DOTA-peptides) and in cases presenting with variable/low SSTR expression.

Multiple tracer imaging, although potentially providing the most accurate biological characterisation of the disease, is not feasible in all patients and should be considered only in selected cases.

7.3 Imaging Protocols

7.3.1 68Ga-DOTA-Peptides

PET/CT acquisition starts at 60 min after intravenous injection of approximately 100 MBq (75–250 MBq) of the radiolabelled peptide (such as 68Ga-DOTA-NOC, 68Ga-DOTA-TOC, etc). The amount of injected radioactivity strictly depends on the daily production of the generator for each single elution (usually ranging between 300 and 700 MBq) and, of course, by the number of patients scanned per day. No specific patient preparation is required (somatostatin analogues treatment should not be discontinued). The use of contrast media is not routinely recommended.

7.3.2 18F-DOPA

PET/CT is performed following the intravenous injection of 5–6 MBq/kg of 18F-DOPA and an uptake time of 60–90 min. It was reported that the oral premedication with carbidopa (100–250 mg, 1 h before image acquisition), a peripheral aromatic amino acid decarboxylase inhibitor, enhanced sensitivity by increasing the tumour-to-background ratio. In particular, carbidopa administration may be useful for the assessment of lesions at sites of increased 18F-DOPA physiologic uptake.

7.3.3 18F-FDG

PET images are acquired after an uptake time of 60 min following the intravenous injection of 370 MBq of 18F-FDG in the 6-h fastened patient.

7.4 Normal Variants, Artefacts and Pitfalls in Image Interpretation

7.4.1 68Ga-DOTA-Peptides

Physiological Biodistribution The pituitary gland, spleen, liver, adrenal glands, head of the pancreas, the thyroid (very mild uptake) and the urinary tract (kidneys and urinary bladder).

Pitfalls [7] False-positive reporting may derive from the presence of accessory spleens, inflammation and lymphoma (due to the presence of SSR on activated lymphocytes and macrophages). Increased tracer uptake at the head of the pancreas is a relatively frequent finding (30–60 %) not necessarily associated with the presence of disease. False-negative findings include small lesion dimensions (<5 mm) and tumours with low or variable expression of SSTR (e.g. medullary thyroid carcinoma, neuroblastoma, insulinoma, pheochromocytoma).

7.4.2 18F-DOPA

Physiological Biodistribution The striatum, adrenals, pancreas and liver with subsequent elimination through the biliary, digestive and urinary tracts

Pitfalls [10] Inflammation (false positive); lesion under the tomograph spatial resolution (5 mm) and low-differentiated tumours (false negatives)

7.4.3 18F-FDG

Physiological Biodistribution The brain, myocardium (variable), liver (low), urinary tract, digestive tract (variable), and muscles (low at rest)

Pitfalls Infection and inflammation (false positives); lesion under the tomograph spatial resolution (5 mm), well-differentiated tumours (false negatives)

Key Points
- 68Ga-DOTA-peptides PET/CT represents the most promising non-invasive imaging procedure to study well-differentiated NEN.
- 68Ga-DOTA-peptides specifically bind to SSTR subtypes overexpressed on NET cells (with variable affinity), but at present, there are no clinical reports supporting the preferential use of one analogue (DOTA-TOC, DOTA-NOC, DOTA-TATE) over the other.
- 68Ga-DOTA-peptides accuracy in NEN lesion detection is superior to morphological imaging procedures, SRS and PET/CT with metabolic tracers (18F-FDG, 18F-DOPA).
- Indications to study NEN include staging/restaging, detection of the unknown primary tumour or of disease relapse, follow-up and assessment of receptor status before PRRT.
- PET/CT with 68Ga-DOTA-peptides has a relevant impact on patient's clinical management (in particular, regarding the choice of the treatment plan) and provides prognostic information.
- 18F-FDG may be useful and provide relevant prognostic information in low-differentiated forms.

- 18F-DOPA is accurate for the assessment of well-differentiated NEN lesions, presenting superior accuracy in comparison to morphological imaging procedures and SRS.
- 18F-DOPA employment is limited by a difficult and costly synthesis and therefore recommended in cases that are not efficiently studied with 68Ga-DOTA-peptides due to variable/low expression of SSTR (e.g. neuroblastoma, pheochromocytoma, medullary thyroid carcinoma).

References

1. Krenning EP, Kwekkeboom DJ, Bakker WH, Breeman WA, Kooij PP, Oei HY, et al. Somatostatin receptor scintigraphy with [111In-DTPA-D-Phe1]- and [123I-Tyr3]-octreotide: the Rotterdam experience with more than 1000 patients. Eur J Nucl Med. 1993;20(8):716–31.
2. Srirajaskanthan R, Kayani I, Quigley AM, Soh J, Caplin ME, Bomanji J. The role of 68Ga-DOTATATE PET in patients with neuroendocrine tumors and negative or equivocal findings on 111In-DTPA-octreotide scintigraphy. J Nucl Med. 2010;51(6):875–82.
3. Schreiter NF, Brenner W, Nogami M, Buchert R, Huppertz A, Pape UF, Prasad V, Hamm B, Maurer MH. Cost comparison of 111In-DTPA-octreotide scintigraphy and 68Ga-DOTATOC PET/CT for staging enteropancreatic neuroendocrine tumours. Eur J Nucl Med Mol Imaging. 2012;39(1):72–82.
4. Gabriel M, Decristoforo C, Kendler D, Dobrozemsky G, Heute D, Uprimny C, et al. [68Ga] DOTA-Tyr3-octreotide PET in neuroendocrine tumors: comparison with somatostatin receptor scintigraphy and CT. J Nucl Med. 2007;48(4):508–18.
5. Ambrosini V, Campana D, Tomassetti P, Fanti S. 68Ga-labelled peptides for diagnosis of gastroenteropancreatic NET. Eur J Nucl Med Mol Imaging. 2012;39 Suppl 1:S52–60.
6. Ambrosini V, Campana D, Bodei L, Nanni C, Castellucci P, Allegri V, et al. 68Ga-DOTANOC PET/CT clinical impact in patients with neuroendocrine tumors. J Nucl Med. 2010;51(5):669–73.
7. Virgolini I, Ambrosini V, Bomanji JB, Baum RP, Fanti S, Gabriel M, et al. Procedure guidelines for PET/CT tumour imaging with 68Ga-DOTA-conjugated peptides: 68Ga-DOTA-TOC, 68Ga-DOTA-NOC, 68Ga-DOTA-TATE. Eur J Nucl Med Mol Imaging. 2010;37(10):2004–10.
8. Koopmans KP, de Vries EG, Kema IP, Elsinga PH, Neels OC, Sluiter WJ, et al. Staging of carcinoid tumours with [18F]DOPA PET: a prospective, diagnostic accuracy study. Lancet Oncol. 2006;7(9):728–34.
9. Kayani I, Conry BG, Groves AM, Win T, Dickson J, Caplin M, Bomanji JB. A comparison of 68Ga-DOTATATE and 18F-FDG PET/CT in pulmonary neuroendocrine tumors. J Nucl Med. 2009;50(12):1927–32.
10. Chondrogiannis S, Marzola MC, Al-Nahhas A, Venkatanarayana TD, Mazza A, Opocher G, Rubello D. Normal biodistribution pattern and physiologic variants of 18F-DOPA PET imaging. Nucl Med Commun. 2013;34(12):1141–9.

Neuroendocrine Tumours Pictorial Atlas

8

Valentina Ambrosini and Stefano Fanti

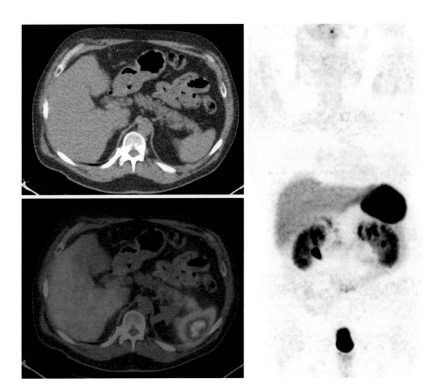

Fig. 8.1 Patient presenting following the incidental detection of a 9 mm nodule at the pancreatic tail. 68Ga-DOTA-NOC PET/CT documented a focal area of uptake (*red arrow*) in the nodule confirming its neuroendocrine nature

Teaching Point 68Ga-DOTA-peptide PET/CT imaging is accurate for the characterisation of even very small well differentiated neuroendocrine lesions.

V. Ambrosini, MD, PhD (✉) • S. Fanti, MD
Nuclear Medicine, University of Bologna, S.Orsola-Malpighi Hospital, Bologna, Italy
e-mail: valentina.ambrosini@unibo.it; stefano.fanti@aosp.bo.it

© Springer International Publishing Switzerland 2016
V. Ambrosini, S. Fanti (eds.), *PET/CT in Neuroendocrine Tumors*,
Clinicians' Guides to Radionuclide Hybrid Imaging: PET/CT,
DOI 10.1007/978-3-319-29203-8_8

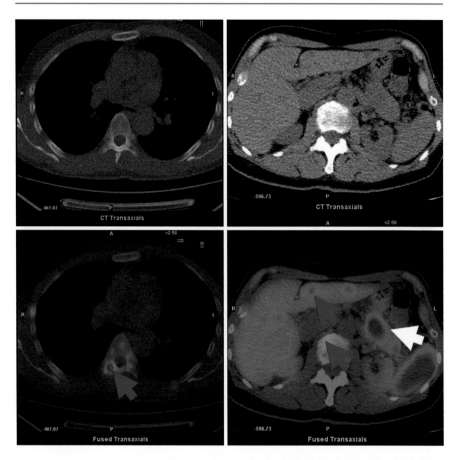

Fig. 8.2 68Ga-DOTA-NOC PET/CT images of a patient studied for staging of a NEN of the pancreatic tail. PET/CT confirmed the primary lesion (*white arrow*) and multiple secondary lesions (nodes, liver, bone; *red arrows*). Pathology on surgical sample documented a G1 disease

Teaching Point PET/CT provides accurate staging (T,N,M) of well differentiated NEN.

Fig. 8.3 68Ga-DOTA-
NOC PET/CT images
showing multiple areas of
tracer pathological uptake
in the left breast (*red
arrow*) of a patient with
multifocal breast NEN

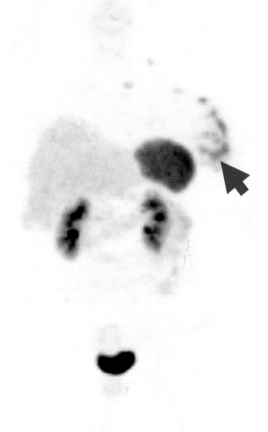

Teaching Point Neuroendocrine differentiation in other solid tumours may occur.
68Ga-DOTA-NOC PET/CT may provide data on SSTR expression.

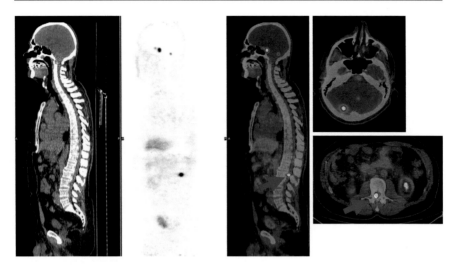

Fig. 8.4 68Ga-DOTA-NOC PET/CT images showing multiple focal areas of tracer pathological uptake (*red arrows*) in a patient with paraganglioma

Teaching Point 68Ga-DOTA-NOC is accurate to study patients with paraganglioma, providing data on somatostatin receptor expression and on disease localization in the whole body.

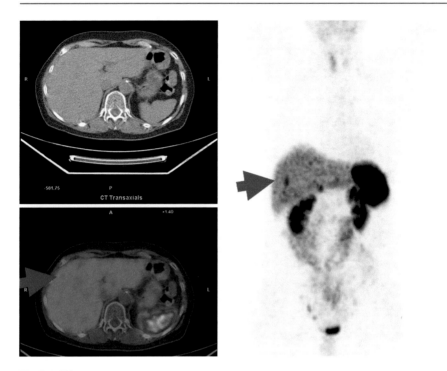

Fig. 8.5 History:
2007: breast carcinoma (surgery + chemo-/radiotherapy).
August 2010: surgical resection of ileum NEN (G2) followed by 68Ga-DOTA-NOC PET/CT (30/09/2010), negative.
The patient was followed up by CT (every 3 months in the first year and once a year afterwards). 2012: at 2 years after primary surgery, CT documented disease relapse at liver level, and 68Ga-DOTA-NOC PET/CT (24/09/2012) showed a focal pathological area at the fifth segment (SUV_{max} = 9, *red arrow*). The patient was addressed to surgical resection of the single liver lesion

Teaching Point 68Ga-DOTA-NOC PET/CT is accurate for the detection of relapse.

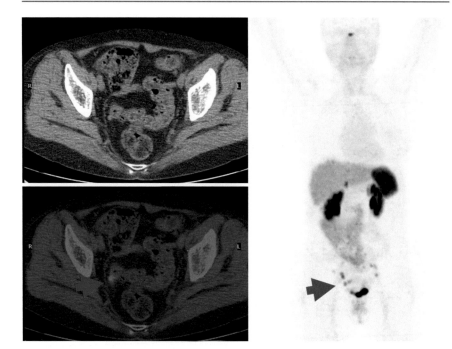

Fig. 8.6 History (same patient as previous image):
2007: breast carcinoma (surgery + chemo-/radiotherapy).
2010: surgical resection of ileum NEN (G2) followed by 68Ga-DOTA-NOC PET/CT (30/09/2010): negative.
2012: relapse at liver level. Surgical resection of the single liver lesion.
2015: After 5 years of the ileal NEN primary tumour resection, a follow-up 68Ga-DOTA-NOC PET/CT showed a multifocal relapse (*red arrows*) undetected by CT

Teaching Point NEN patients may relapse a long time after primary surgery. 68Ga-DOTA-NOC PET/CT can identify relapse undetected by CT.

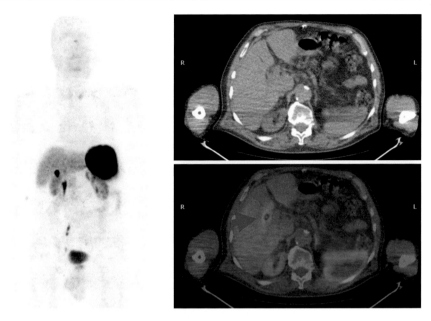

Fig. 8.7 History: patient with HCC, incidental CT-detection (images not shown) of a hypervascularised duodenal nodule of suspicious NE nature. 68Ga-DOTA-NOC PET/CT showed a focal area of tracer uptake of unclear anatomical localization (*red arrow*)

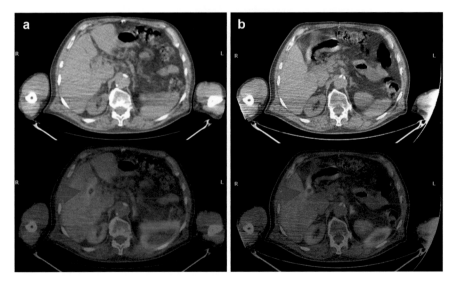

Fig. 8.8 History: patient with HCC, incidental CT-detection (images not shown) of a hypervascularised duodenal nodule of suspicious NE nature.
68Ga-DOTA-NOC PET/CT showed a focal area of tracer uptake of unclear anatomical localisation (**a**, standard 60 min acquisition). Delayed images (**b**) showed a clear projection on the duodenum. *Arrows* indicate sites of disease

Teaching Point 68Ga-DOTA-peptide PET/CT delayed imaging may be useful for better localisation of equivocal imaging findings at standard acquisition time.

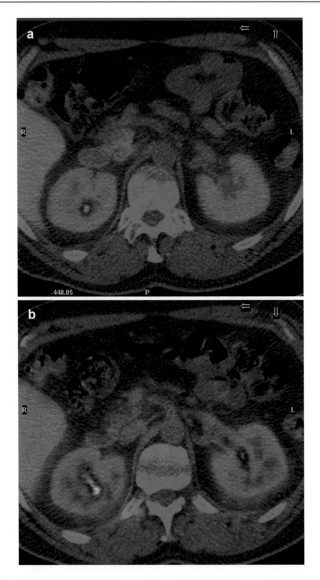

Fig. 8.9 68Ga-DOTA-NOC PET/CT of a patient studied for follow-up of an ileal NET showing a diffuse uptake at the head of the pancreas on one occasion (**a**; February 2009) that disappeared at the subsequent follow-up scan (**b**; June 2009)

Teaching Point Diffuse non-pathologic 68Ga-DOTA-peptides uptake at the pancreatic head may be encountered and may be transient in the same patient.

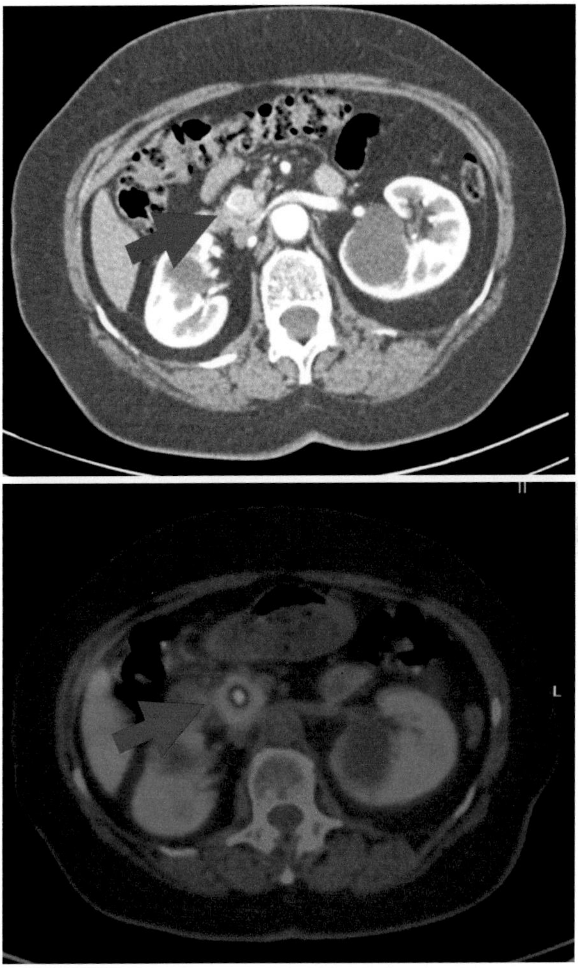

Fig. 8.10 68Ga-DOTA-NOC MIP and transaxial images of a patient presenting with dyspepsia. CT showed the presence of a solid hypervascularised nodule (14×15 mm) at the head of the pancreas. 68Ga-DOTA-NOC PET/CT showed that the nodule presented an elevated expression of somatostatin receptors. *Arrows* indicate sites of disease

Teaching Point Although the head of the pancreas can present a faint diffuse non-pathologic uptake, in the presence of a nodule with increased uptake of the 68Ga-DOTA-peptide, the presence of disease should be suspected.

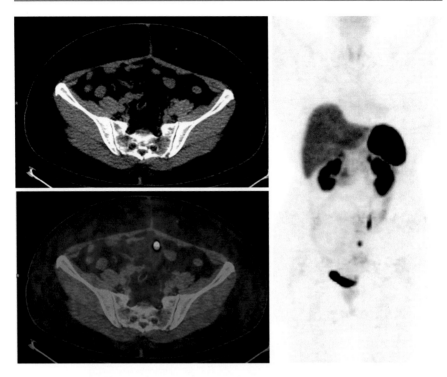

Fig. 8.11 Patient with unknown primary tumour (neuroendocrine tumour assessed on pathology of an excised liver lesion). 68Ga-DOTA-NOC PET/CT documented an area of focal tracer uptake at ileal level suggestive for primary tumour site

Teaching Point 68Ga-DOTA-peptides imaging can be useful to detect the unknown primary tumour site in patients with documented neuroendocrine secondary lesions.

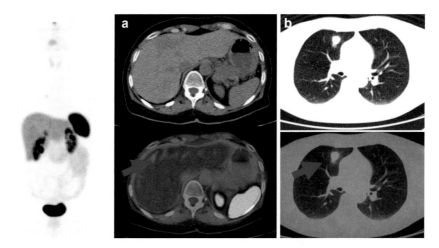

Fig. 8.12 Patient presenting with neuroendocrine liver lesions (G2) but unknown primary site. 68Ga-DOTA-NOC PET/CT showed only faint uptake at bone level (posterior arch of C2, images not shown), while liver lesions were negative (**a**). On low-dose CT images, a lung nodule was detected (**b**). On the basis of these findings, an 18F-FDG PET/CT scan was performed (see next *panel*). *Arrows* indicate sites of disease

Teaching Case In patients with NEN presenting lesions without significant somatostatin receptor expression, 18F-FDG PET/CT should be considered as additional examination.

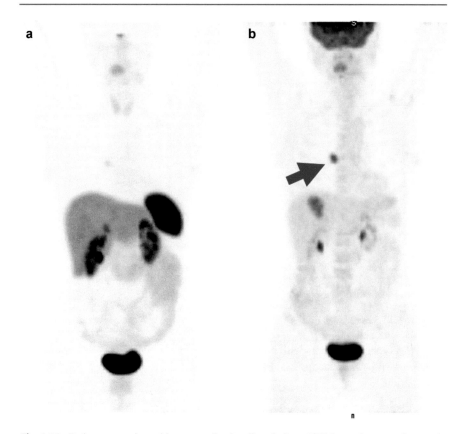

Fig. 8.13 Patient presenting with neuroendocrine liver lesions (G2) but unknown primary site (same patient as previous panel). 18F-FDG PET/CT was performed to evaluate the 68Ga-DOTA-NOC/negative lesions (**a**). 18F-FDG (**b**) documented a hypermetabolic lung nodule (compatible with the primary site; *red arrow*) and metastatic lesions (liver, bone)

Teaching Case In patients with NEN secondary lesions and unknown primary, 18F-FDG PET/CT may provide valuable information on primary site in cases with undifferentiated tumours.

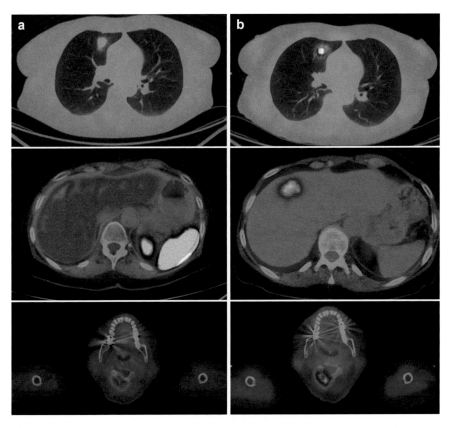

Fig. 8.14 Patient presenting with neuroendocrine liver lesions (G2) but unknown primary site (same patient as previous panel). 68Ga-DOTA-NOC (**a**) and 18F-FDG transaxial images (**b**) comparison. 18F-FDG PET/CT-detected multiple pathological and focal areas of uptake at the right lung (primary) and at liver and bone level

Teaching Point Although generally well differentiated, undifferentiated NET may be encountered, are clinically more aggressive and generally show preferential 18F-FDG uptake.

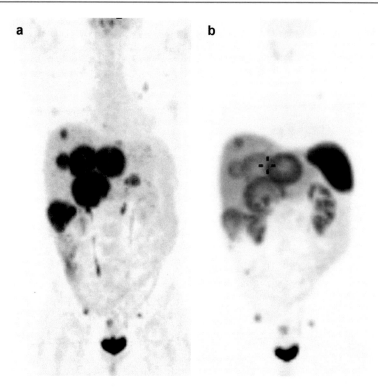

Fig. 8.15 18F-FDG (**a**) and 68Ga-DOTA-NOC (**b**) PET/CT images of a patient with pancreatic (tail) NET with multiple secondary lesions (nodes, liver, lung, peritoneal carcinomatosis) showing some lesions with a cold core area employing both tracers

Teaching Point A cold central lesion area may be encountered in both 68Ga-DOTA-NOC and 18F-FDG PET/CT images, especially in large lesions representing necrosis (in case of concordant findings). It must also be mentioned that in some cases a lesion with a peripheral rim and a cold core at 68Ga-DOTA-NOC PET/CT may present with 18F-FDG uptake only in the 68Ga-DOTA-peptide-negative area; in this case disease differentiation should be suspected.

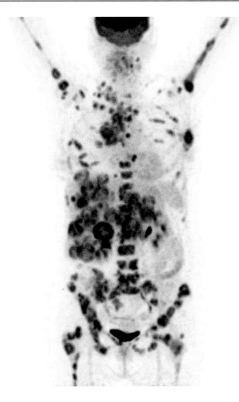

Teaching Point Although most NEN are well differentiated, aggressive forms showing FDG avidity are encountered. High-grade tumours show preferential FDG uptake.

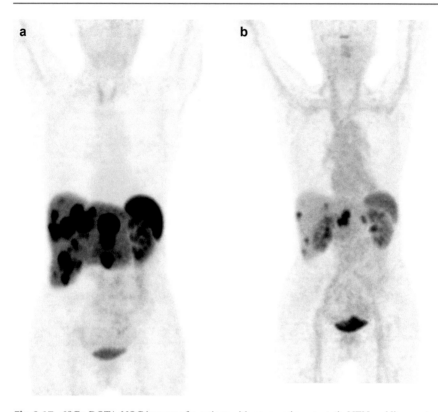

Fig. 8.17 68Ga-DOTA-NOC images of a patient with pancreatic metastatic NEN and liver metastasis studied before (**a**; February 2013) and after PRRT (**b**; September 2013). PRRT induced a reduction in lesions number, size, and uptake (SUV_{max} before PRRT = 37, SUV_{max} after PRRT = 13)

Teaching Point 68Ga-DOTA-peptides uptake correlates with SSTR expression and is useful to select candidate patients for PRRT. 68Ga-DOTA-peptides PET/CT is also useful to guide further treatment planning after PRRT.

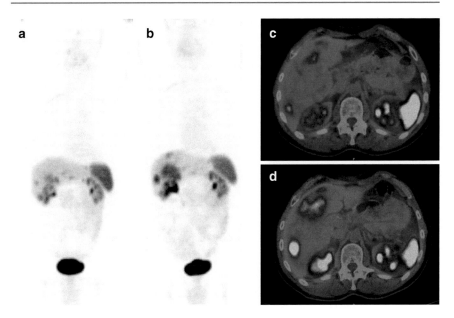

Fig. 8.18 68Ga-DOTA-NOC PET/CT images of a patient studied before (**a**, **c**) and after (**b**, **d**) PRRT showing disease progression

Teaching Point Although ideally a metabolic tracer should be employed to assess disease after therapy, correlating with SSTR expression, 68Ga-DOTA-peptides may be useful to guide further treatment planning.

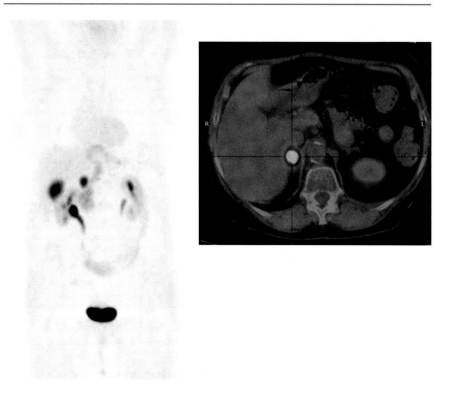

Fig. 8.19 18F-DOPA images of a patient with a clinically suspected pheochromocytoma, showing intense and focal uptake at right adrenal level

Teaching Point 18F-DOPA is accurate for the detection of pheochromocytoma lesions (on the contrary 68Ga-DOTA-peptides have shown suboptimal sensitivity due to the generally low/variable expression of somatostatin receptors)

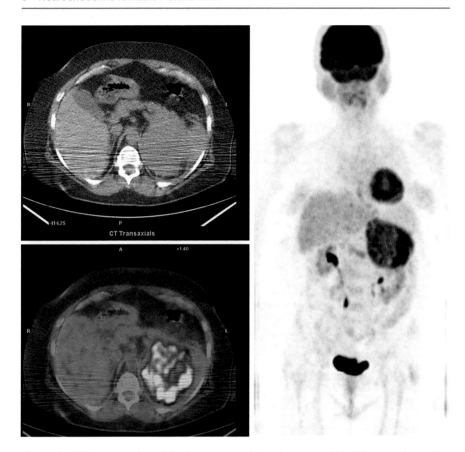

Fig. 8.20 Patient presenting with abrupt onset of otherwise unexplained hypertension and a CT-detected abdominal mass. 18F-FDG confirmed the presence of a voluminous adrenal lesion presenting an increased and heterogeneous uptake ($SUV_{max} = 20$), suggestive for a highly aggressive pheochromocytoma lesion

Teaching Point Although pheochromocytoma may be well differentiated, aggressive undifferentiated forms can be encountered and show a preferential 18F-FDG uptake.

Index

© Springer International Publishing Switzerland 2016
V. Ambrosini, S. Fanti (eds.), *PET/CT in Neuroendocrine Tumors*,
Clinicians' Guides to Radionuclide Hybrid Imaging: PET/CT,
DOI 10.1007/978-3-319-29203-8